Take Me Off the Weight List

Shalynne L. Barr, MBA, CNC

DEDICATION

This book is firstly dedicated to my Lord and Savior Jesus Christ by whom I have been granted life and that much more abundantly. To my husband, Terrence, my best friend, my lover, my biggest supporter. Thank you for believing in me and being in my corner. This book would not have been possible without your encouraging words and prayers. To my sons, Sean and Javon, thank you for all the conversations you allowed me to have just wishing and dreaming about completing this book. Thank you for cheering me on and believing that I could complete it. I am proof that you can do anything you put your mind to.

ACKNOWLEDGMENTS

To all of my supporters, followers and clients, thank you for letting me have a place in your life to awaken your desire to live life with energy and vitality.

To my husband, Terrence and my brother Joshua, thank you for starting the editing process. You got me up and running!

To my best friend Sherita, thank you for letting me talk your ears off the last 13 years about writing this book.

I would be remiss not to acknowledge my Mom, Isha Eefa Williams, who went on before me. It was through her entrepreneurial drive and spirit that I learned firsthand how to make my dreams come true.
This is for you Mom. I will always love you. I miss you tremendously.

CONTENTS

Disclaimer: The information provided is not a substitute for medical care or advice. Information provided is for educational purposes only and is not intended to diagnose, treat, cure, or prevent any disease. Consult your doctor about making diet and lifestyle changes that are right for you.

Interlude 1

Meet Roxy

It was Friday and Roxy had just got off work. She was tired, frustrated and just plain irritated. She trotted down the hall as best as she could and just fast enough to catch the elevator by sticking her thick-footed 3-inch heels in the doorway. Much to her disappointment inside was Hilda and quickly, reality set in that she was going to be taking another icy ride down to the first floor with her again. "How does this keep happening every Friday? I need to find another elevator," Roxy thought to herself.

Hilda was thin, with a body of a Coke bottle, great legs and *everybody* in the building loved her. The only bad thing that Roxy could find on her was her "do-it-yourself" hair weave, which was always crooked in the back. "Somebody really needs to show her how to straighten that thing *out*," Roxy muttered.

Hilda, looked up from her cell phone and pleasantly said, "Excuse? Were you saying something?"

"Oh no, just saying how happy I am to be *out* of the office," Roxy said, "these shoes are killing me."

Hilda looked down at Roxy's feet and could understand why.

Beep...Floor 6. Complete silence.
Beep. Floor 5.
Beep. Floor 4. Hilda sighed contently as she was texting on her cell phone.
Beep. Floor 3. Roxy cleared her throat.

8

Beep. Floor 2. "Almost there," thought Roxy.
Beep. Floor 1. Freedom!

Roxy rushes to the bench to the left of the elevator and sits down to change her shoes. This was her daily ritual. There was no way in the world she could walk all the way to the garage deck in her high heel shoes especially with her back and knees in constant pain. Her doctor told her that she really needed to consider losing some weight.

With her heels now in her shoe bag and her ankle socks and gym shoes on, she was now ready for the hike that was 3 blocks over. Roxy stopped at the corner pastry shop for her normal glazed donut and hot chocolate for her 1-hour ride to pick up Charles Jr., "Chunky Boy," from the daycare. She was a regular and the owner, Paul, always had her treat ready and waiting for her every day at 4:15pm.

Just as she reached her car, she felt the vibration of her cell phone ringing in her pocket. She realized that she had forgotten to take it off of silent when she sat down to change her shoes.

She looked at her cell phone and realized the number was her doctor's office calling. "I wonder why they are calling me? I paid them for my last visit."

"Hello?"
"Hello, Mrs. Constance?"
"Yes, this is she."
"This is the nurse from Dr. Roman's office."
"Yes?"
"We got the results from your blood work test."
"And?"
"Well, we're sorry to tell you that you have diabetes."
"I have what????"

"Yes, ma'am. You have diabetes."

"How is that possible? I added in exercise like the doctor said. I walk every day from my car to the office building in the morning and back to my car when I get off work. Isn't that enough exercise?"

"I'm sorry, Mrs. Constance, I cannot make any comments at this time. Dr. Roman would like for you and your husband to come in for a consultation."

"Ok. I understand," Roxy said, feeling like the wind just got knocked out of her. "Thanks for calling."

"I wish you the best, Ma'am. Have a good day."

Silence on the other end of the cell phone.

1 INTRODUCTION AND MY STORY

Growing up I was not an obese child. I actually was relatively thin most of my life. I didn't have a weight problem. As a matter of fact, I weighed under 100 lbs. until I hit my 20's. In our home, we ate what most folks ate: heavy on the carbohydrates and fried foods (especially fried chicken). Along with that, our main vegetable was corn, which technically is a starch (more carbohydrates!). We typically ate some type of bread or rolls with our meals too and very rarely did we drink water. It was just our way of life. It didn't seem like anything was really wrong with that. The food was delicious and the seasoning was fantastic. But when I look back over those days, I was not eating healthy, well-balanced meals. As I reached my late teens and early 20's and would hang out with my friends more, we would go out to eat. Our favorite places to eat were restaurants called Ram's Horn and Big Boy's. At the time, I was a beef and pork eater so hamburger with fries were my usual choice. I ate so many hamburgers that I'm surprised that I didn't turn into a cow!

At about age 22, things started to change. My poor eating habits finally started manifesting in weight gain. I had graduated from college at Oral Roberts University and I was back home in Detroit. I still was eating out for most of my meals. I started working in Southfield which required me to take three city buses to get there. There was no time for breakfast at all and I was not into packing a lunch, so I usually just bought my lunch at work and dinner was hit or miss. Now with being a younger woman, with not a lot of income to show for, I spent my money haphazardly. "Nutrition" was not a goal of mine and how "healthy" I needed to be was not on my radar. I landed upon an instant favorite: Jiffy cornbread. It was always a main stay in my house right along with all the other breads, but I took it to a whole new level. I would buy Jiffy because I could get 3 boxes for a dollar. Ding! Ding! Right in my budget. Jiffy then turned into my everything for at least a solid year. I know that sounds funny, but I ate more Jiffy then I really care to admit. I always had a fresh loaf on hand. I even would have Jiffy for breakfast. I would crumble it in a bowl and warm it up slightly in the microwave and then add some milk to it. Instantly, I had a mush meal similar to a hot cereal. Delicious.

All that Jiffy, hamburgers, fries and fried chicken landed me an additional 8 lbs. For once in my life I was over 100 lbs. I had finally did it; I broke a threshold of where I had never been before.

I picked up more weight as I moved into my mid-twenties because as I began dating my soon-to-be husband, Terrence, we would go out to eat a lot. It was so much fun to go out to different restaurants around Detroit. But more new restaurants, meant not only the exploration of new foods and more calories too. By the time we were married on December 31, 1994, I weighed 116 lbs. And when Sean was born in 1995, I was a whopping 165 lbs. Wow! I had tipped the scales in my opinion. To this day, I still have stretch marks on my belly and thighs to show for that sudden increase in weight gain. Guess my skin did not know how to react to being stretched so much and so quickly. It's like it exploded.

Like most younger women, quite a bit of my weight fell off after Sean was born, especially since I was nursing. But yet I still carried 15 lbs. of the baby fat that I gained. I rationalized in my mind that I looked ok because now I was "thick" even though I had never in my life been over 100 lbs. I decided it was time to start working off that weight somehow. I started buying VHS tapes and used them to record exercise programs off the TV.

Little Sean would be in his bouncy chair and I would be exercising. Over a small amount of time, I was able to permanently shave off 5 lbs. We then decided to have another baby and along came Javon in 1998. I learned a little bit from carrying Sean though in regards to eating. Reality set in: I could not eat everything in the world. But of course, you know what happened...I still gained a tremendous amount of weight. At the end of my pregnancy with Javon, I weighed about 155 lbs.

I have to say that child-bearing took me by surprise. It was not made known to me that the potential would be there to gain so much weight. As a result, I became depressed. I didn't know what to do with so much excess weight. I had an extra 20 lbs. that I did not want. I did not have consistent time to exercise because my boys kept me busy. As they got older, I ate everything that I fed them including the nuggets and French fries that they loved so much.

Thinking back to those early days, I realize that a sense of defeat and low self-esteem started to rise back up again. Because on a deeper level something in me decided that I was never going to lose the excess weight. And by the time I hit my 30's, my scale had parked itself in the 135 lb. to 140 lb. range. Of course, it did not help that I had not done anything drastically different to combat the weight gain. Now, I will give myself a little credit because I rekindled my love for running from my high school track days and started training for my first half marathon. I still ate poorly during that training though.

As a family, we loved to bake together; that was our bonding time.

13

Quite often the boys and I would make our favorite peanut butter cookies. And, if you know a little bit about me personally, my Mom's homemade caramel corn was definitely made on several occasions for us to enjoy. As far as my nutrition was concerned, I did start incorporating more healthy dishes into our family diet during those days. With my love of reading, the boys and I would go to the library often and get a ton of books. I fell in love with the cookbook aisle.

My outlook on eating really took a turn as a result of one of the cookbooks that I happened to pick up on one of our visits. Unbeknownst to me, it was so much more than a vegetable recipe book. Within the first few pages of the book, I realized that I was on to something. The book that I read talked all about being a vegetarian and about how much animal products we consume in our lifetime and I just about threw up in the library. I remember being stopped dead cold in my tracks.

As a result, in 2004, I became an ovo-lacto vegetarian which excluded meat, fish and poultry but allowed fruit, vegetables, grains, legumes, eggs and dairy, as a result of reading that book. It worked for a while with me seeing a weight decrease of 10 lbs. I was so happy. For the first time in a long time I felt that I was changing things in my life for the better. But with the decrease in my protein level and me not liking the texture of tofu nor the after result of eating beans, my doctor was not happy with the sudden drop in my muscle tone. I found myself back to eating chicken, turkey and seafood in 2006. To this day, I never returned to eating beef, pork and various other types of meats. According to my doctor, due to the length of time that I have not consumed those types of meats, I have lost the enzymes in my body to digest such meats.

For so many years after that I was still on a constant roller coaster both from the nutritional side of things as well as exercise was concerned. I never had a full year where I exercised consistently and ate in a proper manner at once; it was either one or the other. I found myself internally disappointed on a deep level. I began to start sabotaging myself with negative self-talk. I had convinced myself that I could never lose all the weight I had gained over the years. My all-time goal was to get back down to at least 125lbs., which was okay for a then 40-year-old, 5ft. woman. It seemed like a reasonable goal to reach. I just did not have the right tools to do it though. Something was missing.

I went through several desperation phases to get the weight off with using every name brand weight loss program out there. From shakes to home delivered freeze dried meals to point counting systems, you name it, I tried them all.

It wasn't until 2013 that I was completely fed up and disgusted with myself. I started making up little challenges for my friends and I on Facebook. The very first one was called The Natural Soul. For 14 days, we focused on the outside physical body and also on the spiritual side of things too. We learned about the importance of finding harmony in ourselves while learning what it meant to be hydrated.

The next challenge I had was the Power of 7. This one was a little more rigorous. For 7 days, we removed all carbohydrates, ate a large amount of fruit and vegetables only, drank 8 cups of water and exercised for 30 minutes a day.

My mindset was slowly being turned on to this healthier way of doing things and my brain pattern was starting to shift. I also realized that my ideas were helping others too because they were struggling with balance just like me. There was still some work to be done though because even after all of these mini-challenges, I went back to yo-yo dieting.

In January of 2015, I received a shocking report from my doctor. My cholesterol had risen, my white blood cell count level was elevated and I was anemic. That did it for me. I cleaned out my cupboards. I re-adjusted my life and took my quest for good health to social media once again for support. I started a Facebook group called "Eat Clean in 2015." It was a year-long quest to establish accountability for myself and give other people the opportunity to change their eating habits for the better as well. With 123 members, we focused on eating clean foods on a consistent basis.

By mid-summer of 2015, a light bulb turned on in my head to the concept of coaching others. In essence that is what I was already doing. So, the first placed I headed to was the library to find out what did authentic coaching entail. To my delight, I realized that I had enough practical experience through my own experiences and a solid educational basis to begin studying for professional certifications.

I now hold a diploma in Mindful Nutrition and I am a Certified Nutrition Coach (CNC). It is through this education that I am now helping you.

In plain, everyday language, "Take Me Off the Weight List" can help you change your behaviors and mindset to losing weight. It will help you realize that you can lose weight and keep it off. As you read this book you will discover that you have everything you need to lose weight and live a healthy consistent lifestyle. Everything is lying dormant inside of you. Through my personal journey and practical steps, you will be motivated to rid yourself of all the things that have been holding you back. You will no longer categorize yourself as someone who is "trying" to lose weight. You will be known as someone who "did" lose weight. You will be able to finally say, "Take Me Off the Weight List!"

2 GET YOUR MIND RIGHT

As we know, our brain is the centermost being of our nervous system and it is powerful. It wills control over us and declares its power. It is very repetitive in nature in that it will repeatedly perform the same action based upon the habits you have developed. There are countless books in the marketplace that talk about how you are what you think and that you can become a success if you think it. There is truth to those concepts.

Have you ever been around someone who said they just cannot stop watching a certain TV show? Or, they cannot stop shopping at a certain store? Or, maybe they cannot stop eating ice cream? These statements are based upon the "tracks" that have been engraved in their brain. On average, it can take anywhere from 21 to 66 days for your brain to get used to a certain way of doing things and if your favorite TV show is something you watch every day, your brain will automatically tell you when it's time to tune in. The good thing though is that if you have established bad habits they can be broken and new ones can be established.

Stop and think about these brain functions a little deeper. When a drug addict needs help with breaking their addiction they need to be removed from their current environment, right? Can they still visit the drug house regularly and become drug free? Can they be around the drugs that they took on a daily basis and not use those drugs? No. They need to be removed from that environment and put into an environment that is drug free. That is the first step in starting a new pattern.

Your mind controls your thoughts, your actions, your behaviors, and your reactions to people and situations. You decide not to run red lights because an accident can occur. You decide what to wear based upon the style that you have chosen. You decide not to put your hand in fire because you have learned that skin burns. You decide not to drink bleach because it poisons.

Addressing this concept with my clients has been pivotal in my coaching business. Our nutritional backdrop is solely based upon how we associate our thoughts with food. As humans, we have a strong connection to food. We need it in order to survive but what if we ate more from the mindset of being properly nourished versus eating based upon situations, emotions or circumstances? There is a difference between those two aspects.

Just about every event in our lives surrounds itself with food. When someone has a new baby, we take them a casserole. When someone graduates from college we go out to eat after the ceremony. At birthday parties, there is cake. When someone starts a new job, or retires from a job there is a celebration with a meal. At wedding receptions, there is food. At funerals, there is food at the repast and the list goes on and on. Why is there such a strong association with food in our society? In a nutshell, food brings comfort.

We have to be careful though to not trade comfort for imbalance. We have all found ourselves in attendance at one of the aforementioned activities. More often than not the meals that are served are not 100%

nutritionally sound with the proper balance of carbohydrates and nutrients. How does your brain know what to do in these situations? It is going to do what you have trained it to do. For most people that is to eat whatever is in sight.

Let me give you a very liberating statement: You do not have to eat everything that is in front of you. I know that this is a shocker but let me repeat this for you: You do not have to eat everything that is in front of you. Just because you are surrounded by donuts, cake, candy, bread, cookies, pie or pasta, you do not have to eat them. No one is opening up your mouth and shoving food down your throat or at least I hope not! You choose what you put in your mouth.

The question that needs to be addressed now is, how do you make the switch from eating out of habit and for comfort to being more mindful and creating better eating habits?

The same brain that tells you not to run red lights or that tells you not to steal ink pens while on your job, is the same brain that will help you to choose not to eat food that is not good for you. Your brain can even be trained to keep you from eating large quantities of food too even if you grew up in a family where you had to clean your plate before you got up from the table. You have the power to create new habits.

We are a product of our habits, be it good ones or bad ones. Your body responds accordingly. If you feed yourself healthy, nutritious things then your skin is bright, and you are probably lean and toned. You might even get closer to your optimum body weight (notice that I did not say size 0!). Being close to your optimum body weight, gives you a higher capacity to sustain exercising, more energy to play in the yard with your kids and even the ability to go up and down flights of stairs without breathing heavy.

On the contrary though, what does a body that is fed unhealthy food look like? It's probably sluggish, lethargic and has a few aches and pains. The results of eating poorly sometimes shows up in other places of the body too. Sometimes a person's face might have acne, bumps or an outbreak of rashes. Other signs of poor health could be the need for antacids to soothe the digestion process. A continuous diet of unhealthy food can lead to high blood pressure, high cholesterol and even diabetes.

If your mind is geared toward eating unhealthy food, it will continue to think that it needs unhealthy food. But remember that you have the power to create new habits.

If you grew up in Michigan, there were two things that you ate and drank: Better Made potato chips and Vernors pop; no questions asked. I've often wondered what was the secret additive to that potato chip recipe because I could not stop eating them. They are amazingly delicious. I changed this casual love affair of a single serving of potato chips to an on-going addiction. This potato addiction came about because of me. I was the one making myself eat potato chips beyond a lunch time side item. I was the one feeding myself potato chips when I was happy, mad, sad, bored, watching TV or for whatever other reason I could find. I call it an addiction because that is what it really was. That addiction followed me from my teenage years through adulthood and into my marriage.

My husband would try to urge me to eat sweet potato chips as an alternative. They were good but they just were not the same as the regular chips. As silly as this might sound, the close similarity to potato chips would have me crawling back to the actual potato chips because I wanted the "real thing."

Something had to give because I was gaining excess weight from constantly eating potato chips and I knew it but I was in denial because I "needed" my potato chips. I decided that enough was enough. I took these action steps to create a new habit:

A. I acknowledged that I loved potato chips.
B. I acknowledged why I loved potato chips (the smell, the crunch, the flavor and the emotional satisfaction that it gave me.)
C. I accepted that I was gaining extra weight from my obsessive behavior.
D. I admitted to myself that my cholesterol level was out of whack because potato chips have a high cholesterol content.
E. I addressed my emotions as they came and stopped eating out of stress. For example, instead of eating a bag of potato chips to calm me down when I was frustrated, I would thoughtfully and systematically ask myself these questions:
1) What has frustrated me?
2) Why did I allow it to frustrate me?
3) Why did I give that much control to a situation/person and allow frustration to set in?
4) What needs to be done or said to truly resolve this situation outside of eating?
5) If I eat a bag of potato chips does that resolve the situation at hand?

I created this psychological approach to break my addiction. I did not have to get hypnotized, pay a counselor, or tie myself to a tree. I re-trained my thinking to not be driven by my emotions nor eat to find comfort in potato chips.

Walking through this transition was a challenge. It was not easy because just seeing a bag of potato chips was a trigger for me. I remember going to work conferences and they would serve sandwiches and potato chips. Ugh! I was determined to break my addiction though so I made myself not eat what was set in front of me.

I am very proud to say that in 2016, I went 365 days without eating any potato chips. I created new tracks in my brain. I created a new habit. It was a challenge but I did it. Potato chips are no longer a struggle for me. My five-step process worked.

One of the greatest things that you could ever do for yourself is to admit to what you are struggling with. You need to admit the truth in order to help you get your mind on the right track to eating healthy. Some people have every excuse in the world on why they are unhealthy, overweight and why they cannot eat nutritious food or why they do not exercise on a regular basis. For some, it could be because they love to cook and what chef does not eat what they prepare? Some could say it's because "being big runs in our family." Others lean to reasons of "I just don't like to exercise" ... "it's too hard" ... "it's too boring" ... "healthy food is too expensive" ... "I just don't have the time" or "I don't know how to prepare healthy meals." As a health coach, I have heard it all and the excuses could go on forever. But today is a new day! You are reading this book because you are looking for solutions to make some changes in your life and break the addictions that have had you bound, right?

It's time to make some new patterns in that brain of yours. Using my method above, take a few moments and think. Think about what is one or maybe two of the greatest things that you need to change in your eating habits? What addiction needs to be broken? What is stopping you from moving forward? Stop to think about what is blocking you from reaching your health and fitness goal? Is it drinking more water instead of pop? Is it exercising more instead of sitting on the couch for 4 hours a night? Is it eating more healthy foods instead of candy bars? Is it all of these things? I want you to acknowledge that you need to do some things differently to improve your quality of life and that starts with getting your mind right. Not just for the moment so you can get ready for your 20-year class reunion but for a lifetime. You need a lifestyle change.

Let's work through my five-step process together. Take a deep breath to get fresh oxygen flowing to your brain and answer these questions:

1. I acknowledge that I am addicted to (i.e.: eating ice cream, sitting on the couch and not working out, stress eating, hot buttered bread): _____.

2. I acknowledge that I am addicted to this because (i.e.: ice cream is great on a hot summer day; I'm too tired to work out when I come home, stress goes away when I eat, I feel like I'm in heaven when I eat hot buttered bread): _____

   _____

3. I accept that because of my behavior I have gained weight and I am not as healthy as I could be.

4. I accept that because of my behavior, my body has responded with (i.e.: diabetes, high blood pressure, low back pain, acne, being overweight, high cholesterol, retaining fluid in my knees, etc.): _____

5. I am operating out of _____when I give into my addiction? (i.e.: fear, anxiety, anger, frustration)

Now that you have identified *what* is holding you back, let's work on *how* to handle the emotion that is driving you to eat habitually. Use the same word in point 5 from above in point A, B and C below and then answer point D.

A. What has caused _____ in me?

B. Why did I allow my situation to make me feel _____?

C. Why did I give that much control to a situation/person and allow my situation/certain person to make me _____?

D. Outside of emotionally eating, what needs to be done or said to resolve my current situation? _____

   _____

Now write down what your action plan will be going forward. How will you handle triggers as they come? Let's go back to my example of being at work conferences where sandwiches and potato chips were served. I learned that I needed to be prepared with other options of things to eat so I would not give myself the excuse of "there's nothing else to eat so I might as well eat these potato chips." My action plan included 3 main solutions: packing a snack in my work bag, asking the wait staff if they had any fruit that I could have instead of potato chips, or I would even drink an extra serving of water or tea because sometimes hunger can mask itself as dehydration.

In the space below write out your action plan.

1. _____

2. _____

3. _____

4. _____

5. _____

For those of you who live a scriptural-based life, Habakkuk 2:2, says, "Write down the vision and make it plain." It is important to write things down. It will help you define what direction you are headed in. I used my action steps a bazillion times and I have found tremendous breakthrough in my habits and my overall life.

And, if you just completed my five-step process right now, congratulations are in order! You have just taken a huge step towards getting your mind right. Congratulations again!! I am proud of you and you should be proud of yourself too.

One More Thing...

"Once you get your mind right, everything else follows." Anonymous

Interlude 2:

Roxy in Disbelief

Roxy pulled into the daycare feeling numb and in shock to the news that she just received. *"...you have diabetes..."* With the words circling around her head she couldn't wrap her mind around it. How could this be? What would her life be like going forward? All she had ever heard about diabetes is when her Uncle Joe got his toe amputated because of his diabetes. Would that happen to her too? Roxy switched the gear into park and got out the car.

Walking up to Giggles and Wiggles just didn't feel the same in this moment. The normal pep in her step was gone because she had already convinced herself that soon she wasn't going to be able to walk normally any more without all her toes.

Before she put her hand on the front door, Roxy said to herself, "Get it together. Chunky Boy needs you to be happy like how you always are."

"Mrs. Constance!" exclaimed Monique. "How are you today? You're looking lovely as always."
"Thank you", said Roxy hesitantly.
"Are you feeling alright today? You seem like you just saw a ghost or something."
"Oh, I'm fine...I think I'm coming down with the flu or something. I'm just not myself today."
"I can understand that," said Monique. "I was feeling bad myself this morning. But the fog is starting to lift. Let me go see if Charles is ready."
"Ok, thank you."

Chunky Boy was as happy as always whenever Roxy picked him up. He immediately kissed his Mom with a big sloppy kiss as the drool rolled down the side of his mouth when Monique handed him across the counter to Roxy. To this Monique exclaimed, "Aw...he is so cute!"

"Thanks," said Roxy as she managed to get his diaper bag and him balanced on her hip.

Roxy got Chunky Boy all settled in his car seat and he sat down in the front seat. After putting on her seatbelt, she pulled out her cell phone and sent a text: "We need to talk...What time will you be home tonight?"

"8:30pm as always," was the reply.
"I'll put Chunky Boy to bed early."
"Is everything ok?"
"I'm not sure."

3 DON'T WAIT UNTIL YOU GET SICK

As I mentioned at the beginning of my book, the health report I got from my doctor was not healthy at all. My bad LDL's were up, my iron level was low and my cholesterol was high. It was time to make a definitive change and that is what set me on my journey. When I stop to think about it, I needed to be healthy and whole to live a good life for my husband and our sons. What good would I do them if I was sick and unable to move around? If I continued on living in that current state, my poor health could affect them because then I would be dependent upon them to care for me. How was it fair to them for me to live unhealthy? Why would I want them to see me living a life with medications and pills? Didn't I even care enough about myself?

At the time when I was in poor health my body was showing the signs of it. My knees would ache under the extra weight that I carried. My skin would break out. My stomach would be bloated and I would have gas after eating dairy products especially ice cream. I ate a lot of fried food which directly leads to high cholesterol too. But if I knew all these things about myself and I ate them anyway, wasn't I intentionally making myself sick? Was it easier to make myself sick on purpose and deal with the consequences simply because I was undisciplined and I just "had to" eat all my pleasure foods?

27

I allowed my fears of living a consistent healthy lifestyle to paralyze me. I remember being in a frame of mind where I had convinced myself that if I did lose the weight that I would not be able to keep it off, so what was the point?

In my situation, I was making myself sick because of my poor eating choices. This next statement might be controversial but I feel like it needs to be stated: Doctors are not always the answer to your health problems. Sometimes their way of helping is to write a prescription for pills. The true remedy is to address health-affecting problems versus taking a pill to fix everything because what does simply taking a pill really teach you? For the record, I will state that I'm not against doctors or pills but I'm definitely all about getting to the root of issues. Pills are like band-aids in my opinion.

Today is your day to make a choice. Not tomorrow. Not five minutes from now but in this moment right now you need to decide that you want to be healthy and you want to be fit. Decide that you want to change the quality of your life before some type of sickness arises.

Change is good and I understand that change can sometimes be scary but when change is going to lead to positive results then it is necessary. How do you face the fear of change? How can you make a 180° turnaround from how you are currently living? The amazing thing about fear is that when you face it, you realize that it is not as bad as you thought it was. Zig Ziglar stated that "fear is False Evidence Appearing Real".

At some point in our lives we all face fear. You might have faced fear when jumping off the diving board for the first time or maybe standing up in front of a crowd and giving a speech. Or, maybe it could have been going through culinary school and presenting your dish to the head chef for a full rating. There is always a point in time where you have to face your fear and decide that you are going to overcome the fear that has you bound.

What if your fear of making healthy changes has kept you in a crazy loophole? What if your fear of stepping on the scale to see how much you weigh has kept you from losing weight? Sometimes, we sabotage ourselves and our minds can trick us into thinking, "It's not that bad" or that "You can lose weight at any time". But what if the damage is severe enough that you have to lose weight? That's the point where I was at; I had to lose weight because I was making myself sick.

So as not to be so one-sided, sometimes some factors truly can be out of our control too. Let's consider another reason why people should pay attention to what they eat: allergies. Being allergic to certain foods can cause you to be sick. If you think you are getting sick from what you eat, please pay special attention to this section.

The Food and Drug Administration (FDA) has a Big 8 list. This list is comprised of foods that typically make people sick because of their reaction to them.

The eight foods are:
Milk
Eggs
Fish (e.g., bass, flounder, cod)
Crustacean shellfish (e.g., crab, lobster, shrimp)
Tree nuts (e.g., almonds, walnuts, pecans)
Peanuts
Wheat
Soybeans
Source: http://bit.ly/2fv13d2

My friend Tina found a way to determine what foods were possibly making her sick. Here's her story:

"For my entire adult life, the muscles in my neck and back were very tight. At times, I would have to turn from the waist to look at something as I could not move my neck without a lot of pain. I used to joke that my back was so tight you could drive a car over it. Due to the tight muscles, I also had a problem with headaches. A friend told me I might have an intolerance to something in my diet causing inflammation. She had recently gone on an elimination diet and suggested I try it. I spoke with my massage therapist who agreed that this could be a likely cause of my muscle tightness.

I started an elimination diet right before Thanksgiving. Most people would have waited until after the holidays but I was determined to do anything I could to feel better. I brought my own food to Thanksgiving dinner at my sister-in-law's house. I was stuffed and satisfied. I had a little twinge of remorse for missing out on the foods others were eating but not much because I was already starting to feel better and healthier. While most people were gaining weight, and feeling sluggish during the holiday season, I was losing weight, feeling great and had energy. I hadn't been working out but I felt like I had a coiled energy just like when I had been regularly running.

Through the elimination diet, I learned I had an intolerance to dairy. When I reintroduced dairy, I immediately had digestive issues, nausea, a headache, and body aches. If I had continued to eat dairy I would have gotten over those issues but the intolerance would have manifested once again in my muscles. With the dairy, out of my system, my massage therapist said that she could see my shoulder blades for the first time and the headaches caused by my tight muscles were gone. Some exercises that had made my arms go numb were now not a problem. I also lost 20 pounds while on the diet. I have continued to avoid dairy, eat healthy and as a result I feel great!"

I, like Tina, discovered my own food reactions but I kept eating food from those food groups anyway. One of my main issues is dairy; I am lactose intolerant. Although dairy is extremely beneficial to our bodies since it supports our calcium level and gives us strong teeth and bones, I still allowed myself to suffer from the aftereffects of it on my body. Wildly enough, I was comfortable with being sick.

Finally, after suffering many years from stomach cramps, flatulence and being bloated, I had to move away from dairy and find another way to get the calcium support that I needed. I found that support in kale, broccoli and spinach.

Our bodies can be very forgiving and resilient. It can moderately function with the presence of adverse and non-ideal conditions but there is always a breaking point. There is a point where your body starts to show signs that something is out of whack. Do not wait until you are sick to change your lifestyle. Listen to your body now. What is it saying to you?

I believe in good stewardship. Webster defines stewardship as the activity or job of protecting and being responsible for something. Stewardship is also a biblical concept where we are to be in good management of what we have been entrusted with just like the parable in the New Testament about the young man and the ten talents.

I Corinthians 6:19-20 even speaks about how our body is the temple of the Holy Spirit and how we should honor God with our body. Once I realized that I was failing in this area, this scripture totally revamped my life. I am a woman of faith and because I believe in God, I want to follow the principles in the Bible even the ones that talk about how our faith and fitness go hand in hand. I'll explain more about that in the next chapter.

When I was born on July 1, 1971, I was in great health. I was free of ailments. I did not have high cholesterol. I did not have low iron. I was a picture of good health. As an adult, I moved away from that good health. How did that happen? As a baby, I was not fed fried chicken and mashed potatoes. I was fed foods that would help nourish my organs and help me to grow. At some point, I became responsible for my own food choices and so did you.

31

Take an introspective look at yourself. What have you done to yourself since you became old enough to choose your own food? Have you taken good care of yourself? Have you been a good steward of what you have been given? Your body is a direct result of how you treat it. What you put inside yourself, manifests on the outside. You *show* what you eat.

Since the basis of eating healthy is dependent upon what we eat, how do you choose what style of eating to follow? There are several eating styles to follow. Many will say that eating all protein is the way to go. Several feels that cutting all carbohydrates out of your diet is the answer and still there are others that swear by eating a complete raw diet and yet others eat according to their blood type. After following so many of these ways of eating styles personally, nothing has been as beneficial to me as eating clean foods.

Clean eating, in my opinion, is one of the simplest and most nutritious ways of eating. It yields to much flexibility and variety. There is no calorie counting and no measuring. Following this line of eating mainly entails being mindful of where your food originates from and how you prepare it. Our bodies crave all natural, healthy unprocessed food and clean eating fulfills that need. For more recipes and how to get started with clean eating check out my companion e-book, "Clean Eating for People on the Go."

There are 7 basic principles to clean eating:
1. Eat food in its healthiest state by limiting processed foods. This means eating food as close as possible in its natural state. If you eat broccoli, for example, do not drown it in heavily processed cheese sauce. Simply steam it and season it with a dash of pink Himalayan salt and black pepper. Or, if you like chicken, do not fry all the nutrients out. Consider sautéing it in olive oil or coconut oil. You would be amazed at how much more flavor you can taste and how delicious it is.

2. Limit sugars. According to the American Heart Association, the maximum amount of added sugars you should eat in a day are a lot less than what the average person consumes on a regular basis. Men: 150 calories per day (37.5 grams or 9 teaspoons). Women: 100 calories per day (25 grams or 6 teaspoons). Unfortunately, sugar does not add any nutritional value to us at all. It contains no vitamins or minerals. It is technically a carbohydrate. It can be habit forming too. Check out http://bit.ly/2jZMQGJ for more information on sugar consumption.

3. Reduce salts. The FDA recommends between 1,500mg and 2,400mg per day. If you have a diet that is hefty in processed foods, you are more than likely at that limit in just one meal. Pay attention to what you are eating; there is salt in everything. Ranch dressing typically has 260mg per 2 Tbsp. and even a glass of milk has 130mg. Excess salt in your body raises blood pressure and can put you at risk for a heart attack or stroke.

4. Eat more vegetables. The advantages of this food group are so extensive that I could fill up two chapters alone just talking about it! Vegetables provide the fiber that is needed to keep your digestive system moving. With being rich in vitamins and minerals they can help you feel full too. Vegetables help to reduce the risk of chronic diseases and can improve the health of your eyes possibly preventing cataracts. Be mindful of starchy vegetables such as potatoes and limit your intake. You could never eat too many green leafy vegetables like spinach, lettuce, Swiss chard and mustard greens. Aesthetically speaking, vegetables add vibrancy and color to your plate.

5. Increase your fruit intake. Fruit helps to correct the deficiencies of vitamin A and vitamin C. Folic acid; fiber and potassium are also nutrients that your body needs and you can get that from fruit. Eating more fruit can help reduce the

risk of kidney stones and help to strengthen your bones against osteoporosis as you get older. Many of the berries are especially beneficial: blueberries, strawberries and even cranberries. Add in citrus fruits as well. Eat all fruit in their natural state and not dried. Dried fruit is loaded with added sugar. To minimize your caloric intake, limit your fruits to about 1-1/2 to 2-1/2 cups per day.

6. Eat whole grains and reduce the amount of refined flours. Whole grains help reduce the risk of heart disease and contains fiber that can keep you from being constipated. Whole grains are great when it comes to helping to manage your weight because they help keep you full. Explore other grains; try something different. I have fallen in love with millet and barley.

7. Reduce food items that are manufactured with refined flours. It's very simple...stay away from processed foods like cookies, cakes, cereals, white rice and white pasta.

If fear was not an issue for you to make your necessary lifestyle changes, would you move forward? If you could dispel the self-doubt of "I'm not capable of being healthy on a consistent basis" or "I know I can't keep the weight off", would you make the change to live a healthy lifestyle? I think you would and now is your opportunity. Let's kick fear in the butt!!!

Fear Elimination Worksheet

1. If you were to take a snapshot of your current state of health, what would you say is the greatest area that needs to be addressed?

_____

2. What fearful thoughts have you had that have kept you from addressing the areas that need to change?

_____

3. If you do not face your fears and address what needs to be changed in your current state of health, what types of medical conditions could develop?

_____

4. Close your eyes and imagine what good health looks like for you. Describe it in full detail below.

_____

_____

5. In your personal life what was the last tough situation that you faced and conquered?

_____

6. What steps did you take to conquer that situation?

_____

_____

_____

7. Apply those same steps to facing your fears about changing your current state of health for the better.

_____

_____

_____

If you answered these questions thoughtfully and was very honest with yourself, you should be able to see that what is blocking you from achieving good health is really not fear at all. It is your mindset. If you have been able to conquer fear and reach tough situations in other areas of your life, you can do the same when it comes to your health.

In the space below, write down a new daily affirmation that you can tell yourself. Write down what your new mindset will be from this day forward.

Complete this sentence. Today is a new day! I will see myself as a person who is...

_____

_____

_____

One More Thing...

"The best part about changing your life for the better is that you have the power to actually do that. You have the capability to improve the quality of your life and live a healthy life." Shalynne Barr

4 FAITH AND FITNESS

My life is rooted and grounded in my faith and I stay focused on my health and fitness journey because of it. For me, the two go hand in hand and cannot be separated. In fact, I did an in-depth study in the Bible and found several scripture passages that related to HOW and WHY one should take care of their body.

At a minimum, it takes 21 days to make a habit. Well, I took that literally and I identified 21 scriptures that helped me along my journey to good health. I stood upon these scriptures to give me encouragement and strength on days when I felt like I could not do another rep on my weights or when I felt like I was about to jump into a bowl of ice cream and do back strokes.

To follow are the scriptures that I identified as key scriptures and my commentary on how I applied the scripture to my life. Under "What does this scripture mean to you", write how the scripture impacts you and how you can apply it to your life. All scriptures are quoted from the New Living Translation.

My hope is that these scriptures will bring encouragement to you and strengthen your faith while you are on your journey to living a healthy, balanced lifestyle.

37

Scripture 1:

Deuteronomy 30:19-20

Vs. 19: "Today I have given you the choice between life and death, between blessings and curses. Now I call on heaven and earth to witness the choice you make. Oh, that you would choose life, so that you and your descendants might live!"

Vs. 20: "You can make this choice by loving the LORD your God, obeying him, and committing yourself firmly to him. This is the key to your life. And if you love and obey the LORD, you will live long in the land the LORD swore to give your ancestors Abraham, Isaac, and Jacob."

What does Health Coach Shalynne think about this scripture? You can choose life today by focusing on your health and eating properly.

I love how this passage also makes a point and speaks about our descendants. That's talking about our children and grandchildren. What kind of example are you being before them? They are watching you and they look up to you. Be a good example.

Choose life!

What does this scripture mean to you?

_____

_____

_____

Scripture 2:

Proverbs 14:1

"A wise woman builds her home, but a foolish woman tears it down with her own hands."

What does Health Coach Shalynne think about this scripture? Many have read this scripture and thought about it from the aspect of the physical house that we live in. The thinking was that if a woman is mean, angry, disrespectful and unloving, her family life would be destroyed thus the breaking down of her house with her bare hands.

But remember that your natural body is your house too. You live in your body. You can tear that house down with your bare hands by what you feed yourself. You use your hands to eat, right? So, if the food that you are feeding yourself is beneficial or non-beneficial becomes a matter of your choice.

Will you choose to tear down or build up your house today?

What does this scripture mean to you?

_____

_____

_____

Scripture 3:

2 Samuel 22:30

"In your strength, I can crush an army; with my God, I can scale any wall."

What does Health Coach Shalynne think about this scripture?
Without God's strength, we cannot do anything. We are rendered powerless without Him. We need Him in our lives.

When it comes to eating, I have had all kinds of food addictions beyond potato chips; I was a junk food junkie. As I've mentioned before, I got to a place where I knew that things had to change. I also began to realize that I could not fight this war on my own. I needed God on my side. I needed Him to show me how to be freed from these food addictions that had me bound. Being able to break down these walls was the key to good health and I knew that but I could not do it on my own.

I needed Him to fight for me. I needed Him to help me fight against my army of addictions and replace my bad habits for healthy ones.

Now I am free!

What about you? What walls are standing in the way of your good health? Pray and ask God to help you kick down any barriers that you might have in your life.

Good health is on the other side of that wall!

What does this scripture mean to you?

_____

_____

_____

Scripture 4:

Philippians 3:13

"No, dear brothers and sisters, I have not achieved it, but I focus on this one thing: Forgetting the past and looking forward to what lies ahead."

What does Health Coach Shalynne think about this scripture? What if you just accepted your past way of doing things and learned from it? What if you no longer walked in defeat and condemnation? How would your life be if you lived according to honoring God in your body daily?

Don't be bound by your past. This is the purpose of this book! Turn off that little cassette tape that is playing these negative words in your head:

1. You can't do this for more than 2 weeks
2. You are a failure
3. There's no way that you can ever reach your goal weight
4. This might be good for now but you cannot survive the holidays

Tell that voice in your head to shut-up! Accept your past. Learn from it and move on! Press on towards the better days that are ahead. You got this!

What does this scripture mean to you?

_____

_____

_____

Scripture 5:

1 Corinthians 9:27a

"I discipline my body like an athlete, training it to do what it should..."

What does Health Coach Shalynne think about this scripture? Your body can only do what you make it do. It will not do jumping jacks on its own. It cannot do sit-ups on its own. And it definitely cannot feed itself unless you do it.

The key word in all of these sentences is YOU. You are responsible for training your body.

Will you choose to train your body well?

What does this scripture mean to you?

_____

_____

_____

Scripture 6:

<u>1 Corinthians 10:13</u>

"The temptations in your life are no different from what others experience. And God is faithful. He will not allow the temptation to be more than you can stand. When you are tempted, He will show you a way out so that you can endure."

<u>What does Health Coach Shalynne think about this scripture?</u> This scripture is perfect for the weekends. Most weekends are full of birthday parties, baby showers, dinner dates, family gatherings and at all of these events are 100% organic foods, right?? WRONG! All kinds of sweets, cookies, cakes, rich breads and butters will abound for sure.

Prayer has worked the best for me when I am faced with temptation to eat something that is less than beneficial. I stop and quietly pray and ask God to help me overcome what my mind is screaming at me to eat. Works every time!

<u>What does this scripture mean to you</u>?

_____

_____

_____

Scripture 7:

<u>Ephesians 2:10</u>

"For we are God's masterpiece. He has created us anew in Christ Jesus, so we can do the good things he planned for us long ago."

<u>What does Health Coach Shalynne think about this scripture?</u> These words should jump out at you. You are God's Masterpiece. That means that you are beautiful. You are a work of art. When something is exquisite how is it treated? Do you deface it? Do you destroy it? Pieces of art are quite often handled with pure, white, clean gloves.

How do you treat the body that God gave you? Are you treating yourself as the Masterpiece that it really is?

<u>What does this scripture mean to you</u>?

_____

_____

_____

Scripture 8:

Ephesians 6:10

"A final word: Be strong in the Lord and in his mighty power."

What does Health Coach Shalynne think about this scripture? It's a new day and you have a fresh set of days ahead of you. Learn from each milestone that you have taken and improve upon what areas need tweaking. If you worked out only two times last week, this week work out three times. If you only drank four cups of water per day last week, this week drink five.

But no matter what, don't you dare do this in your own strength. Trust in the Lord and lean upon Him for strength. He is there for you.

What does this scripture mean to you?

_____

_____

_____

Scripture 9:

<u>1 Corinthians 6:19-20 NLT</u>

"Don't you realize that your body is the temple of the Holy Spirit, who lives in you and was given to you by God? You do not belong to yourself, for God bought you with a high price. So, you must honor God with your body."

<u>What does Health Coach Shalynne think about this scripture?</u> God gave us our bodies. We are His. He has entrusted us to take good care of our temples so we must honor Him. How do we honor Him in our bodies? By eating healthy, nutritious food and exercising.

This scripture has been the key to the consistency of my journey. I want to please God according to all His principles in the Bible and not pick and choose which scriptures to obey. This one in particular always hits home for me and is a constant reminder of how I should be caring for my body. I feel that this scripture has helped me not to gain back the weight that I loss and it has also helped me not to go back to binge eating potato chips.

<u>What does this scripture mean to you</u>?

_____

_____

_____

Scripture 10:

Psalms 37:5

"Commit everything you do to the LORD. Trust him, and he will help you."

What does Health Coach Shalynne think about this scripture? People sometimes forget that God gives us the ability to choose. We choose our actions, patterns and disciplines. He gifted us with the capacity to make choices.

Commit to increase your faith in God to help you live a consistent healthy lifestyle. Choose good health. After that choice has been made, your next step is to simply trust Him to help you stand firm with that decision.

What does this scripture mean to you?

_____

_____

_____

Scripture 11:

Proverbs 3:7-8

"Don't be impressed with your own wisdom. Instead, fear the LORD and turn away from evil. Then you will have healing for your body and strength for your bones."

What does Health Coach Shalynne think about this scripture?

Sometimes our own rationale can lead us astray. We can convince ourselves that we really don't "need" to exercise or that we don't really "need" to drink water. Don't be deceived by your own negative self-talk.

Be encouraged to turn to the Lord for wisdom on how to live a healthy lifestyle. When you do, you will have good health in your body.

What does this scripture mean to you?

_____

_____

_____

Scripture 12:

<u>**Daniel 1:5**</u>

"The king assigned them a daily ration of food and wine from his own kitchens. They were to be trained for three years, and then they would enter the royal service."

What does Health Coach Shalynne think about this scripture? This passage speaks to discipline and focused concentration. In the Bible, the Hebrew boys had nutritional structure in how they ate and they also had a fitness plan.

Meal planning and exercise plans have been the foundation to my journey. This type of consistency and structure can yield great results just like it did for the Hebrew boys. The scripture says that at the end of their training period, they were entered into royal service. What a great reward.

Your reward of good health can be just as great! Get started now.

What does this scripture mean to you?

_____

_____

_____

Scripture 13:

Psalms 139:13

"You made all the delicate, inner parts of my body and knit me together in my mother's womb."

What does Health Coach Shalynne think about this scripture? God knows everything about our bodies because He created us. Why not lean upon Him for wisdom when it comes to living in good health and being fit?

I am an avid knitter and what stands out to me from this scripture is how He "knit" us together in the womb. In knitting, you have to pay attention to the pattern or your item will come out lopsided and not wearable. God cares so much about us that He has carefully crafted and fashioned us. Now it is our responsibility to take care of what He has given us.

What does this scripture mean to you?

_____

_____

_____

Scripture 14:

Proverbs 23:2a

"If you are a big eater, put a knife to your throat;"

What does Health Coach Shalynne think about this scripture? This scripture stopped me in my tracks when I first read it. In my heart, I don't believe that God is honored when we gorge ourselves. Overeating is an addiction. The tell-tale sign that you are suffering from overeating is when you are not able to control yourself and you eat whatever you want, whenever you want and how much you want.

Use this affirmation to conquer overeating:
Food no longer has a grip on me. I use my food as fuel for my body so I can be healthy, fit and strong. I will not use my fork as a weapon to overindulge. I can control how much I eat because I can do all things through Christ who gives me strength!

What does this scripture mean to you?

_____

_____

_____

Scripture 15:

Romans 7:15

"I don't really understand myself, for I want to do what is right, but I don't do it. Instead, I do what I hate."

What does Health Coach Shalynne think about this scripture? This scripture speaks directly to discipline within ourselves. There is a war waging within you: the right thing to do vs. the wrong thing to do. Will living a healthy, balanced life prevail? The choice is yours.

What does this scripture mean to you?

_____

_____

_____

Scripture 16:

1 Corinthians 10:31
"So, whether you eat or drink, or whatever you do, do it all for the glory of God."

What does Health Coach Shalynne think about this scripture? It doesn't get much clearer than this!

What does this scripture mean to you?

_____

_____

_____

Scripture 17:

Proverbs 25:27a
"It's not good to eat too much honey..."

What does Health Coach Shalynne think about this scripture? I read this scripture to mean that there is a warning in regards to eating too many sweet treats. Also, take notice that it does not say never to eat them. The scripture just says that it is not good to eat too much honey.

Desserts and sweet treats are the biggest area that most people struggle with and it has derailed many from their quest for good health. Learn to put parameters around how much sweets you can have. I typically recommend one sweet treat a week.

All things in moderation.

What does this scripture mean to you?

_____

_____

_____

Scripture 18:

Psalms 30:2
"O LORD my God, I cried to you for help, and you restored my health."

What does Health Coach Shalynne think about this scripture? I'm hoping that since the start of this chapter you are taking time to pray and ask the Lord for help to break down the barriers in your life that have caused you not to focus on your health.

From this scripture, it is clear that if you call out to God and ask Him for help, your health can be restored and set on a journey to be healthy and balanced. Isn't that fantastic? Amen! God desires for us to be healthy and I want you to be healthy too.

What does this scripture mean to you?

_____

_____

_____

Scripture 19:

Ecclesiastes 9:7
"So, go ahead. Eat your food with joy, and drink your wine with a happy heart, for God approves of this!"

What does Health Coach Shalynne think about this scripture? Before you freak out and think I'm telling you to get turnt up on wine, I want you to re-read this passage again. Food was designed by God and we should enjoy it and use it for its proper usage: to fuel our bodies and help us live a healthy lifestyle.

There is one word that I want to highlight: JOY! This scripture conveys just that. Be joyful about living a healthy lifestyle. The rewards that you will reap are amazing!

What does this scripture mean to you?

_____

_____

_____

Scripture 20:

3 John 1:2
"Dear friend, I hope all is well with you and that you are as healthy in body as you are strong in spirit."

What does Health Coach Shalynne think about this scripture? In this scripture, John is writing to his friend Gaius. There are some good points in this short passage:

1. John cared for his friend.
2. John wanted his friend to be healthy so could it be possible that Gaius needed some encouragement along his health and fitness journey?
3. Accountability is key.

Who are you accountable to? Connect with a friend today.

What does this scripture mean to you?

_____

_____

_____

Scripture 21:

Psalms 107:20-21

"He sent out his word and healed them, snatching them from the door of death. Let them praise the LORD for his great love and for the wonderful things he has done for them."

What does Health Coach Shalynne think about this scripture? Just as this scripture states, the word of God can heal us. Our health can be revived from a dead, dormant state to a lively state of wholeness and well-being.

Be healed today from past mindsets that have held you captive. Be set free in knowing that God loves you and through His word you can have life and that much more abundantly.

What does this scripture mean to you?

_____

_____

_____

It is my hope that after studying these 21 scriptures from the Bible that you can see how much God loves you and cares about all aspects of your life including your health and your fitness level. Through Him and the Bible, your faith should be strengthened and you should have a better understanding on how to use scriptures in times when you feel weak along your journey to obtain good health.

Be encouraged today in knowing that God is on your side and through Him you can live life with energy and vitality.

One More Thing...

Proverbs 3: 5-6 NLT: Trust in the Lord with all your heart; do not depend on your own understanding.

Interlude 3:

Roxy in Denial

"Well, we're sorry to tell you that you have diabetes."
These words just kept clouding her head and ringing in her ears. How could this be? Roxy knew that she needed to make some minor changes to her health but she never imagined that her current state of health was so poor that now she had a name for it. She never wanted to be "labeled" as having anything. And diabetes of all things? Her thoughts were interrupted with the precise 8:30pm jiggle of Charlie's keys in the front door.

Roxy turned away from washing dishes and dried her hands. When their eyes met he saw that something wasn't right.

"Angel face, what's the matter? What's going on?" as he set down his lunch bag on the table.
"I got a call from Dr. Roman's office today."
"They got the results from your test?"
"Yes, and they must have my information mixed up with someone else."
"What do you mean? How is that possible? What did they say?"
"They said I have diabetes."
Silence.
Tears begin to slowly roll down Roxy's face as the pinned-up emotion from those words, *"Well, we're sorry to tell you that you have diabetes,"* re-played through her head again.
Charles held her close as her body shook violently. He didn't let her go and together they stood in the kitchen left to wonder how their lives were going to change going forward?

5 FEED ME!

Your body trusts that you will take good care of it. You are its main resource for sustenance. It has no other way to get its proper nutrition, well maybe through an IV, but you know what I mean. You have the sole responsibility of feeding yourself properly on a daily basis. Before I took this responsibility seriously, my daily diet used to look something like this:

Breakfast: Turkey bacon, oatmeal and decaffeinated coffee with sugar and flavored cream
Morning Snack: Granola bar and a caramel Frappuccino
Lunch: Spicy chicken sandwich combination with fries and strawberry-lemonade
Afternoon Snack: Potato chips
Dinner: Fried chicken, prepared box rice/pasta, vegetables and cornbread
Evening Snacks: More potato chips or homemade cookies or *maybe* some fruit

For many years, I ate like this. I actually thought it was acceptable to eat whatever I wanted. I did not look at things from a big picture standpoint. I was not considering how my poor eating habits were affecting my body internally. I was "happy" because in essence I was feeding my emotions. It was a vicious cycle and deep down inside I was not truly "happy"? The results from eating whatever I wanted began to leave some evidence. My clothes were getting tighter. I didn't have the energy that I needed to go up and down the stairs in my house. I felt lethargic. My body was talking to me. It was telling me that I was doing something wrong. It was telling me that I needed to make some changes and fast!

Our bodies have a baseline that it should not cross and it is called homeostasis. The word homeostasis means being balanced. We are in proper balance when we eat healthy, nutritious foods and when we minimize our sugar and carbohydrate intake. When an improper balance in homeostasis is present, the cells in our body begin to perform in a different manner thus causing our insulin to spike. The body begins to become sluggish and more commonly that sluggishness is found after eating a heavy, non-nutritious meal.

Let's look back at the example of how I used to eat. My old way of eating definitely caused my body to lose its homeostasis. How does this compare to how you eat normally? Write in what a normal day looks like for you.

Shalynne's Old Way of Eating	*Your Daily Eating Routine*
Breakfast: Turkey bacon, oatmeal and coffee with sugar and flavored cream	Breakfast:
Morning Snack: Granola bar and a caramel Frappuccino	Morning Snack:
Lunch: Spicy chicken sandwich combination with fries and strawberry lemonade	Lunch:
Afternoon Snack: Potato chips	Afternoon Snack:

Dinner: Fried chicken, prepared box rice/pasta, vegetables and cornbread	Dinner:
Evening Snacks: More chips or homemade cookies or *maybe* some fruit	Evening Snack:

Take a moment to reflect. How does your normal day of eating look to you? Is it anything close to my old way of eating? Let's start with today. What have you eaten so far today? How much processed food have you eaten in comparison to clean foods? How much fruit have you had? How much water have you had?

Now it's time for some homework! Yup, that's right. For the next seven days, I want you to track what you eat and I mean everything. From that morning English Muffin for breakfast to that evening bowl of ice cream. And don't try to alter anything. Be honest! The truth starts with you and it starts today.

You need to see what you are eating. The proof is in the pudding. (Well, maybe that's not a good food choice for my example, but I think you get what I mean.) It's time for you to look at what you are actually feeding yourself. The point of this exercise is not to condemn you but it is to help you know what food groups you need to add to your eating habits and which ones you need to minimize or eliminate altogether.

In the pages ahead, I have included my simple-to-use 7-Day Food Tracker Log. Use this tracker to log your food. Take special note of what time you are eating your meals too; that is important. You will also need to log how much water you drink each day. After your seven days of tracking, we will do an analysis of your data. You will be able to score yourself.

Seven Day Food Tracker Log

Day 1

Today's Date: _____

Breakfast: (Time: _____) _____
_____

Snack: (Time: _____) _____

Lunch: (Time: _____) _____
_____

Snack: (Time: _____) _____

Dinner: (Time: _____) _____
_____

Snack: (Time: _____) _____

Additional Food Eaten: (Time: _____) _____

End of the Day Wrap Up:

Daily Totals	Fruit	Carbohydrates: Cereals, Breads, Grains, Beans, Rice	Vegetables	Water (How many 8 oz. cups did you drink?)
How many servings did you have today? For example, if had two pieces of fruit then you would write in 2.				

65

Seven Day Food Tracker Log

Day 2

Today's Date: _____

Breakfast: (Time: _____) _____
_____

Snack: (Time: _____) _____

Lunch: (Time: _____) _____
_____

Snack: (Time: _____) _____

Dinner: (Time: _____) _____
_____

Snack: (Time: _____) _____

Additional Food Eaten: (Time: _____) _____

End of the Day Wrap Up:

Daily Totals	Fruit	Carbohydrates: Cereals, Breads, Grains, Beans, Rice	Vegetables	Water (How many 8 oz. cups did you drink?)
How many servings did you have today? For example, if had two pieces of fruit then you would write in 2.				

Seven Day Food Tracker Log

Day 3

Today's Date: _____

Breakfast: (Time: _____) _____
_____

Snack: (Time: _____) _____

Lunch: (Time: _____) _____
_____

Snack: (Time: _____) _____

Dinner: (Time: _____) _____
_____

Snack: (Time: _____) _____

Additional Food Eaten: (Time: _____) _____

End of the Day Wrap Up:

Daily Totals	Fruit	Carbohydrates: Cereals, Breads, Grains, Beans, Rice	Vegetables	Water (How many 8 oz. cups did you drink?)
How many servings did you have today? For example, if had two pieces of fruit then you would write in 2.				

Seven Day Food Tracker Log

Day 4

Today's Date: _____

Breakfast: (Time: _____) _____

_____

Snack: (Time: _____) _____

Lunch: (Time: _____) _____

_____

Snack: (Time: _____) _____

Dinner: (Time: _____) _____

_____

Snack: (Time: _____) _____

Additional Food Eaten: (Time: _____) _____

End of the Day Wrap Up:

Daily Totals	Fruit	Carbohydrates: Cereals, Breads, Grains, Beans, Rice	Vegetables	Water (How many 8 oz. cups did you drink?)
How many servings did you have today? For example, if had two pieces of fruit then you would write in 2.				

Seven Day Food Tracker Log

Day 5

Today's Date: _____

Breakfast: (Time: _____) _____
_____

Snack: (Time: _____) _____

Lunch: (Time: _____) _____
_____

Snack: (Time: _____) _____

Dinner: (Time: _____) _____
_____

Snack: (Time: _____) _____

Additional Food Eaten: (Time: _____) _____

End of the Day Wrap Up:

Daily Totals	Fruit	Carbohydrates: Cereals, Breads, Grains, Beans, Rice	Vegetables	Water (How many 8 oz. cups did you drink?)
How many servings did you have today? For example, if had two pieces of fruit then you would write in 2.				

Seven Day Food Tracker Log

Day 6

Today's Date: _____

Breakfast: (Time: _____) _____
_____

Snack: (Time: _____) _____

Lunch: (Time: _____) _____
_____

Snack: (Time: _____) _____

Dinner: (Time: _____) _____
_____

Snack: (Time: _____) _____

Additional Food Eaten: (Time: _____) _____

End of the Day Wrap Up:

Daily Totals	Fruit	Carbohydrates: Cereals, Breads, Grains, Beans, Rice	Vegetables	Water (How many 8 oz. cups did you drink?)
How many servings did you have today? For example, if had two pieces of fruit then you would write in 2.				

Seven Day Food Tracker Log

Day 7

Today's Date: _____

Breakfast: (Time: _____) _____
_____

Snack: (Time: _____) _____

Lunch: (Time: _____) _____
_____

Snack: (Time: _____) _____

Dinner: (Time: _____) _____
_____

Snack: (Time: _____) _____

Additional Food Eaten: (Time: _____) _____

End of the Day Wrap Up:

Daily Totals	Fruit	Carbohydrates: Cereals, Breads, Grains, Beans, Rice	Vegetables	Water (How many 8 oz. cups did you drink?)
How many servings did you have today? For example, if had two pieces of fruit then you would write in 2.				

Seven Day Food Tracking Summary

7 Day Total	Fruit	Carbohydrates: Cereals, Breads, Grains, Beans, Rice	Vegetables	Water (How many 8 oz. cups did you drink?)
Tally up all your servings for the week and put them in the appropriate column.				

Let me explain a couple of things before we start reviewing your data. Through bio-individuality, we all have significant differences in anatomy and physiological parameters but as a rule of thumb, you should follow the 80/20 rule. Make healthy food choices at least 80% of the time and give yourself a 20% variance and eat foods that are semi-less than nutritious. Note that when you eat something that is not the most nutritious, it takes your body 8-12 hours to regain its homeostasis balance. Ultimately, we want to nourish our bodies on a consistent basis to thrive and not just to survive.

Let's look closely at each food category and determine how they should properly fit within our everyday eating patterns.

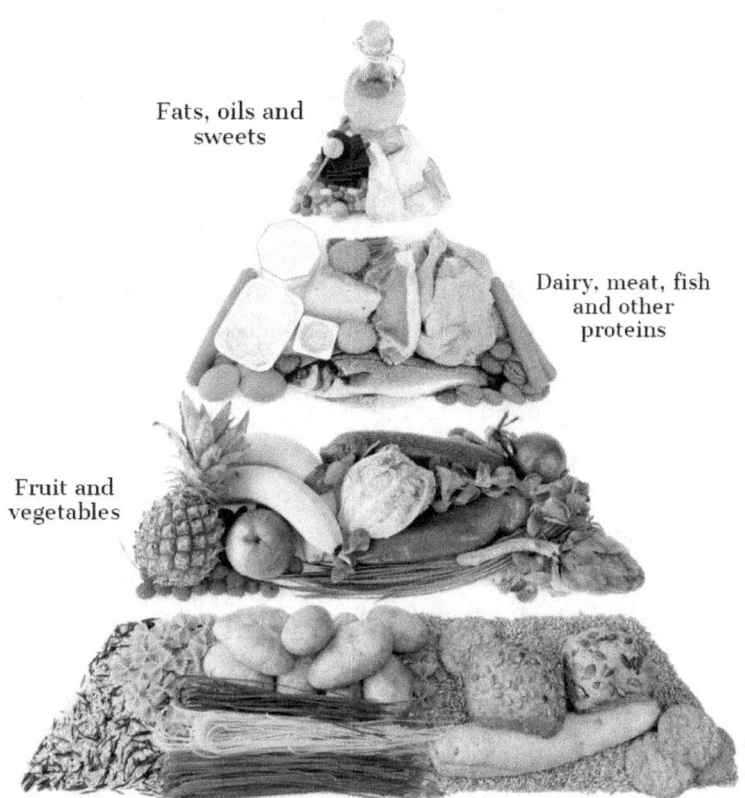

Fats, oils and sweets

Dairy, meat, fish and other proteins

Fruit and vegetables

Bread, grains, beans, pasta and other starches

<u>Fats, Oils and Sweets (use sparingly):</u> There are two main types of fats: healthy fats and unhealthy fats. Steer clear of the unhealthy fats such as saturated fats and trans fats. They are more commonly found in fried foods and desserts. Replace butter, gravy and most commercial salad dressings with healthy fats such as olive oil, coconut oil, grapeseed oil and even avocado oil. Be mindful of the amount of sugar that you are eating. Use healthy alternatives such as dates and monk fruit extract to sweeten your dishes and drinks.

<u>Milk and Yogurt (2-3 servings daily):</u> Many people grew up hearing, "Milk does a body good." Yes, milk does build strong teeth and help supports our bones and as we age it does help to prevent osteoporosis because of its calcium content but limit your servings to 2-3 per day to minimize fat intake. Babies and children need much more in their formative years but even as they get older they do not have to have as much either. Choose yogurts such as Greek yogurts and those that do not have sweetened fruit added to it. Try out cottage cheese. Several vegetables are rich in calcium too such as kale, spinach and broccoli.

Meat, cheese, fish, eggs and other protein (2-3 servings daily): Although quality protein is vital to health and healing, the average American consumes beyond the amount of protein that is needed daily. Excess protein is stored as fat. Consume between ½-1 gram of protein per day for every pound of lean body weight. Also, distribute protein evenly throughout the day to help with the enzyme functions of the body. Meat, cheese, fish and eggs are the more commonly known sources of protein but other meatless options are: pea protein, quinoa, beans and almonds/almond butter.

Fruit (2-4 servings daily): Fruit is an excellent source of vitamin A and C. Be careful of eating canned fruits that have been sweetened with corn syrup. Remember: Fresh is best. A quick solution to adding more fruit to your diet is to eat fruit that comes in a form that you can quickly grab; no utensils required. Apples, oranges, bananas, pears, plums, grapes and blueberries are all great options.

Vegetables (3-5 servings daily): "Eat your vegetables" is what I grew up hearing my Mom say. Vegetables are so beneficial but sometimes this category is non-existent in people's lives. Your body needs vegetables to get folic acid and magnesium since it cannot produce it on its own. For clients that cannot stand the sight of vegetables, I offer these suggestions: juice them in a juicer and drink them; grind them in a food processor and mix them in your meatloaf or spaghetti sauce; or add a handful of kale or spinach in your morning smoothie. Eating a variety of vegetables will help you get the phytonutrients that you need thus boosting your immune system.

Breads, grains, cereals, rice, beans and pasta (6 servings per day).
Your body needs fiber to aid your digestive system's daily functions.
Even though this food grouping provides this, it also has the
propensity of becoming addictive and yielding the highest level of
"comfort food" options. To combat overeating and to help maximize
nutritional value, take careful consideration in your selection. Be
conscious of your bread choice. Choose whole wheat, millet or chia
bread over white bread. Select brown rice over white rice. Create your
own whole wheat pasta dish with minimal and delicious ingredients
over the prepared mixes that are laden with salt, butters and
saturated fats.

Now let's look back on your 7 Day Food Tracking Summary and let's
compare them to what is recommended for us. Copy your numbers
again below.

Your Seven Food Tracking Summary

7 Day Total	Fruit	Carbohydrates: Cereals, Breads, Grains, Beans, Rice	Vegetables	Water
Tally up all your servings for the week and put them in the appropriate column.				

If we were to total up the maximum amount of recommended servings that you should have per week from all the food groups, it would look something like this:

Recommended Weekly Servings per the USDA

Weekly Allowance	Fruit	Carbohydrates: Cereals, Breads, Grains, Beans, Rice	Vegetables	Water (Based upon 8 cups a day)
These numbers represent the maximum amount of servings you should typically eat within a week.	28	42	35	56 cups

What do you think? How are you measuring up to the recommended daily allowance? To the recommended weekly allowance?

_____

_____

What food groups do you need to eat more from? _____

_____

What food groups do you need to eat less from? _____

_____

How about your water intake? What was the highest amount of water you drank in one day? What was the lowest amount? _____

Again, as previously stated, the purpose of this exercise and these questions are to help you better understand your current eating habits. Maybe your findings were great and you were pleased with your tracking. Congrats to you. Great job! Maybe you found that there was room for improvement. That's ok too. Just make a conscious decision to change your eating habits for the better.

I know firsthand the happiness that comes with choosing healthy things to eat and as an end result having more energy and vitality. I want you to experience that same feeling and you can. It all starts with your food choices.

One More Thing...

"How willing you are to make changes is directly dependent upon how motivated you are to get where you want to go." Crystal Paine

6 WATER

All lifeforms depend on water. Besides oxygen, water is the next important nutrient. Water is vital to our overall health and well-being. The body can only go approximately 3 days without water. Without water, you would not survive. Your lungs are 90% water. Your brain is about 95% water. Your bones are 25% water. Your blood is 82% water.

With normal everyday activities, you lose water and that water needs to be replaced. By drinking water, you help to replenish your bodily fluids. We become thirsty when our water level decreases even slightly and begin to experience dehydration. Even a 2% drop in water level can trigger dehydration. This small drop in water level can result in dry skin, loss of appetite, chills, and even elevated cholesterol. "Estimates indicate that approximately 75% of Americans have mild, chronic dehydration." (Source: NAFC Trainer, pg. 108)

To keep your body at a normal range of hydration, you should drink half your bodyweight in ounces on a daily basis. A 170lb. person should drink 40 oz. per day plus an additional 6-12 ounces per every 15-20 minutes of exercise. How does your daily water intake compare to this rule of thumb?

Dehydration can show up in many ways besides just feeling thirsty.

1. Bad breath: If you are not drinking water, the saliva in your mouth can sit and become fermented. Bacteria begins to grow and causes bad breath.
2. Fatigue: The lack of water causes your blood pressure to drop, your heart rate to increase, and blood flow to the brain slows down. With the increased work of these major muscles you feel tired and fatigued.
3. Muscle cramps: Although more commonly seen in athletes during sporting events, cramping is a byproduct of dehydration. When a low level of hydration is detected in the body, organs shift fluid away from the least important area at the time to protect itself. More often than not muscle cramps show up in legs.
4. Headaches and dizziness: Our brain responds negatively to the lack of water, resulting in an inability to focus, dizziness or feeling foggy.
5. Constipation: The body removes water from your colon causing your stool to be harder and firmer. Drinking more water can aide in making it easier is to eliminate.

Water also helps you to consume less calories because of how full you feel when you drink it. I suggest having a glass of water about 30 minutes before you eat and I always suggest water over diet drinks even the zero calorie ones. Nothing replaces the benefits of pure water.

Let's not overlook the connection between water and the function of our kidneys. Our kidneys remove toxins from our body. You need water in your system for this to happen though. "Through the posterior pituitary gland, your brain communicates with your kidneys and tells it how much water to excrete as urine or hold onto for reserves," says Guest, who is also an adjunct professor of medicine at Stanford University. http://wb.md/2hwDOME

Those reserves help to keep the body operating properly, no matter if you drink water or not (to be honest). The body will always protect its major organs first. But when it detects that there is just barely enough water to function, your brain will trigger that the water threshold is in jeopardy and that is when you begin to feel thirsty.

The biggest problem that I hear from clients when they start drinking water consistently, is that they have to go to the bathroom all the time. I totally understand that! But that's a good problem to have. Remember, using the bathroom dispels toxins.

There is technically no set time that you have to drink water but there are times that can be more beneficial than others. For example, drinking water in the morning helps to wake up your system and can cause you to eliminate the food from the night before. Drinking water in the afternoon can give you energy.

I like to plan out my daily water intake. I have a bottle of water in the morning while I am working out. I will get another bottle in mid-morning. Another bottle around mid-afternoon and then on the way home from work I'll drink another bottle. Following this type of plan helps my body to stay at an even hydration level all day. Now, I have to admit, I am getting just a little older (just a little) so I cannot drink a lot of water before going to bed. So, at max, I need to get all my water for the day in by at 8:00pm.

If you think that water is bland and just horrible, you can jazz it up a little bit without compromising its health benefits. All you need is a water bottle with an infuser in it.

Here are my seven favorite infused water combinations:

1. Cucumber-Mint
2. Strawberry-Lemon

3. Lemon-Lime
4. Pineapple-Mint
5. Lemon-Orange
6. Blueberry-Grapefruit
7. Apple-Cinnamon Stick

Here are several other recipes to infuse your water:

1. Pineapple-Strawberry
2. Cherry-Lime
3. Blueberry-Orange
4. Watermelon-Basil
5. Pineapple-Orange
6. Strawberry-Lime-Cucumber
7. Lemon-Cilantro
8. Kiwi-Cucumber
9. Watermelon-Mint
10. Lemon-Raspberry-Rosemary

To make these combinations, simply wash the fruit/vegetables/herbs. Slice or dice them and put them in the infuser. Place the infuser in the water bottle and add water. I usually use purified water. I enjoy my infused water chilled so I prepare my infused water at night and put it in the refrigerator so it's ready to go in the morning. The longer you infuse, the more robust the flavor. Give some of these a try or make up your own. Experiment and get creative!

Once I became an avid water drinker, I noticed several differences in myself. My nails were stronger, my hair grew faster, my skin cleared up and started glowing.

The health benefits of drinking water are wonderful and quite beneficial...drink some water today!

One More Thing...

"Water is the only drink for a wise man."
David Henry Thoreau

7 EXERCISE

In order to lose weight, you have to exercise. It is through exercising that you burn calories thus weight loss occurs. Sounds simple enough, right? Well, in our ever-busy lifestyle and beyond demanding schedules, exercising sometimes falls low on the to-do list. But just like anything else in your life, if you make it a priority you can find time to exercise.

I know all too well the struggle of making time to exercise on a consistent basis. My normal pattern was to exercise "here and there". Even my favorite types of workouts (cardio aerobics, kickboxing and weightlifting) was not enough to sway me into consistency. I remember times where I had a complete exercise plan created and even my workout clothes laid out for in the morning. But if I woke up late or had a slight change in schedule, I would not exercise at all.

What does inconsistency or "yo-yo exercising" do to the body? Starting and stopping can potentially be more detrimental than not exercising at all. Being inconsistent, puts your body at risk and can even lead to muscle damage. You can also experience sore muscles, stiffness, muscle fatigue, loss in stamina and muscle tone.

Back in my inconsistent days, I did not find the value in exercising regularly. I had fifty million excuses that I thought were valid. I used to have a relaxer in my hair before I locked my hair in Sisterlocks and my hair was my biggest excuse: "My hair is going to get messed up with all that sweat" and even "My curls are going to flatten out."

I used to blame the equipment that I had at the time too. The old treadmill that I had did not calibrate right, so I felt that I could not get an adequate reading of my exercising so I would not workout. It was really loud too. I remember saying that I did not want to wake anyone up that was sleeping so I could not exercise. Didn't my family need to sleep peacefully after all? One excuse after another kept me from exercising consistently.

One day I sat down and described all my different phases of exercising and created fictional people who carried my traits. While they are quite humorous, I wonder if you could find yourself to be similar to these people or carry a little bit of their personalities?

Let me introduce you to my friends.

"Pre-meditator Peter":
Peter is the type of exerciser who has thought about exercising several times. He has purchased DVD workout plans, dumbbells and even gym memberships. The DVD's are so precious to him that he uses them as coasters on his coffee table. Peter has an extensive fitness wardrobe including yoga pants, dry fit tank tops, headbands and the new cooling cloths that cool you off for hours. He constantly talks about how quickly he can get back into shape and how he is just waiting until after he comes back from his vacation to get started again. Peter usually makes his upcoming workout plan while on his vacation so when he gets home he's ready to get started.

"Beginner Betty":
Betty cannot count the numerous amount of times that she has started and stopped her exercise plans. She has completed all types of exercise plans dating back to Richard Simons and Jane Fonda. Betty is one step ahead of others because she will at least begin a workout plan. The funny thing about her though is that she has never completed a full program! She has printed off several plans from the

Internet: weightlifting, yoga, Pilates and even Tai Chi. Betty starts them all but she quits easily. Several times she has even stopped mid-session in the workout because she was "tired." Betty knows that she should do more but she is on this roller coaster ride that she cannot get off of.

"Let's Rock this Larry":
Larry is the man! He has been exercising consistently for a year. He has lost 32lbs. since he changed his eating habits and added in exercise consistently. Without fail, he is in the gym every week for one hour on Tuesday, Thursday and Friday. He takes his multi-vitamins daily and never runs out of his whey protein mix. Larry has toned, tightened and chiseled every inch of his body and is now focusing on his calves because they still seem a "little puny". He has that ever coveted 6 pack, is sporting the "Y" cut at his waist and has finally developed the "horseshoe" on the back of his triceps. When he is at the gym everyone stops and stares because he just looks fantastic. Larry follows a specific diet and has no room for junk food or cheat meals. Larry actually is considering becoming a certified nutrition coach because he has seen phenomenal results for himself.

"Superhuman Harriett":
Have you seen Superhuman Harriett lately? Oh my! She has rock hard abs and biceps as big as cantaloupes. She works out twice a day and has zero body fat. She is a vegetarian and eats all organic fruits and vegetables. She recently quit her corporate job so that she could go into full time body building and get her certification in personal training. When she is with her clients, friends and family, she is the picture of good health but Harriett secretly loves donuts and brownies. When she is alone she eats them and she eats a lot of them. Harriett has slipped into binge eating and has lost track of how to live a healthy, balanced life.

Although these profiles are fictional, they may be a reality for some people because they were for me. Can you find yourself closely related to one or two? Or, a mixture of two? What can you do to remove the traits that you do not like and create new ones?

Probably to your surprise, this chapter is not going to lay out a full blown, step-by-step workout system. The purpose of this chapter is to help you think. I want you to identify what is keeping you from exercising consistently. I want you to uncover your excuses and determine if they are truly valid. You really don't need another book to give you an exercise plan. Exercise plans can be found everywhere. You need help with understanding that the exercise plans cannot work without you. You need to work the plan.

How do you find the motivation to exercise regularly? How do you turn the corner to finally say that I am going to exercise on a daily, weekly, and consistent basis from month-to-month and year-to-year?

It has to go beyond just saying, "I am going to do it." You've said that before. That doesn't work, right? You have to take action.

Here are 5 ways to keep yourself motivated to exercise:
1. Reward yourself! For every pound that you lose put $5 in a jar. Once you get to a certain milestone during your weight loss journey, go buy yourself a beautiful dress or a new pair of slacks. Maybe the first clothing item comes after you lose 10 lbs.; that would be $50 that you have earned!!
2. Grab a friend. There is nothing like the accountability of a true friend. A friend will be there to motivate you, to encourage you and to push you on days that you don't want to work out. If you both have similar goals, then you will both be losing weight in no time.
3. Jump on the Internet. There are online workout clubs, online programs and even apps. Quite a few plans also allow you to set up reminders. The reminder can chime at a certain time every day and that will keep you on track. I provide online programs for my clients; they love them and have seen great success.
4. Use your TV as a motivator. Do you find yourself getting home from work and sitting on the couch for 4 hours until it's time to go to bed? Use your time wisely and exercise on the commercial breaks. On average, each commercial break is about 2 minutes. In 2 minutes, you could do between 20-25

jumping jacks or 40 crunches or maybe 30 push-ups. There is so much that could be done in just 2 minutes.

5.   Be accountable to yourself. Keep an exercise journal. I have written down every exercise that I have done since the beginning of the year. Having my journal helps me keep a visual track record. Even on days that I do not work out, I write down why I did not work out that day. I love this form of accountability.

In order to lose weight, you must burn more calories than you are consuming. To follow is a chart to help you drill down how many calories you can potentially burn when you exercise.

Calories Burned During Activities

Approximate calories burned per hour *All numbers are estimates and will vary based on weight, body composition and intensity level.					
Activity	**100lb. person**	**125lb. person**	**150lb. person**	**175lb. person**	**200lb. person**
Aerobics, Step: high impact	480	600	720	840	960
Aerobics, Step: low impact	336	420	504	588	672
Aerobics: High impact	336	420	504	588	672
Aerobics: Low impact	264	330	396	462	528
Aerobics: Water	192	240	288	336	384
Basketball: Wheelchair	312	390	468	546	624
Bicycling, Stationary: Moderate	336	420	504	588	672
Bicycling, Stationary: Vigorous	504	630	756	882	1008
Bicycling: 20 mph	792	990	1188	1386	1584
Bicycling: 12-13.9 mph	384	480	576	672	768
Bicycling: 14-15.9 mph	480	600	720	840	960
Bicycling: 16-19 mph	576	720	864	1008	1152
Bicycling BMX/Mountain	408	510	612	714	816
Bowling	144	180	216	252	288
Boxing: Sparring	432	540	648	756	864
Calisthenics: Moderate	216	270	324	378	432
Calisthenics: Vigorous	384	480	576	672	768
Chopping/Splitting Wood	288	360	432	504	576
Circuit training: General	384	480	576	672	768
Dancing: Disco, ballroom, square	264	330	396	462	528
Dancing: Fast, ballet, twist	264	330	396	462	528
Dancing: Slow, waltz, foxtrot	144	180	216	252	288
Elliptical trainer: General	432	540	648	756	864
Gardening: General	216	270	324	378	432
Golf: Carrying clubs	264	330	396	462	528
Golf: Using cart	168	210	252	294	336
Gymnastics: General	192	240	288	336	384
Handball: General	576	720	864	1008	1152
Heavy Cleaning: Car, windows	216	270	324	378	432
Hiking: Cross Country	288	360	432	504	576

Source: http://bit.ly/2yDdhF7

What is the point of this chart? Pick an exercise and get going! You cannot afford not to exercise.

Now, it's your turn. Let's create an action plan. Without a plan, you will just be spinning your wheels (which is actually a form of exercise!) Plan out your week. Look at each day in your upcoming week and find 30 minutes that you could exercise on at least 4 days of the week. This is your time to do something for yourself. Get creative. You do not have to exercise at the same time every day either. Maybe one day you have to work in the evening so consider exercising first thing in the morning. Grab a simple calendar and create your plan. Post it on your fridge and put your plan to work.

You will also need to track your progress along the way. Weigh yourself before you start your plan. Please do not drive yourself crazy with weighing yourself every day though. Excessive weighing in will set you up for disappointment in part because your body fluids fluctuate from day to day, thus causing your scale to go up and down. Best practice is to pick a certain day to weigh in and jot down the day and the weight at that time. Also, track your body measurements with a measuring tape. No matter what the scale says, the measuring tape is always accurate.

Exercising is important to your health. Add some today!

One More Thing

"Strength doesn't come from what you can do, it comes from overcoming the things you once thought you couldn't do." Rikki Rogers

8 YOU CAN DO IT!

One of the biggest advantages to being healthy and being fit is that once your overall health improves you feel great. I want you to experience a life of freedom and happiness that comes along with a healthy, balanced lifestyle. You deserve to live with energy and vitality. If nothing else stands out to you from this whole book, I want you to remember these four words: "YOU DESERVE GOOD HEALTH!"

Losing weight is like achieving any other goal that you have set your mind to do. Did you decide to go to college and get a degree? Did you decide to save money and buy a car? Did you decide to adopt a rescue dog? Did you decide that you wanted to take a vacation to Hawaii? Did you decide that you wanted a promotion on your job and you started working later hours and shadowing the boss? Did you decide that you wanted to mentor abandoned children so you signed up as a foster parent?

What about the simpler, everyday things? Did you decide to brush your teeth this morning? Did you decide what color carpet you wanted in your basement? Weren't you able to decide what kinds of rules that your children were to abide by? Aren't you capable of meeting deadlines that your boss asks you to fulfill? And how about choosing your outfit for the day?

My point is that when you decide to do something you actually do possess the willpower and the strength to do it, right? You are capable of doing so many things and so why not choose to lose weight and be healthy on a consistent basis?

I have perfected some of my Mom's and my Grandmother's most prized recipes. They taught me well. But with this being said, I have decided that I cannot make batches of caramel corn, key lime pie or 7-up pound cake on a regular basis. This would not be a wise decision. Why? Because I would eat it all!! There is a place for these favorite treats in my life but not every day. I reserve these delicious family desserts for special occasions. That's a decision I made and I have stood by this decision.

The same with you. You must know your limits and limitations. If your trigger food is chocolate covered pretzels, enjoy them every other week and not every day. Do you love pop? Can't live without your favorite coffee? Then make it apart of your plan but just not every day.

Put it this way: if your food or drink obsession is not a healthy benefit to you, it needs to be minimized and not maximized in your life. Are there grey lines to the aforementioned statement? Probably. I'm sure someone could say that coffee is good for you because it helps to get your system going, but what about all the added sugar and cream? Is that healthy too? We know that zucchini is good for you but what about when it is fried or even made into chocolate zucchini cake?

Let's talk about priorities. I finally got to a place in my life where I had to own my adulthood and make smart, wise and positive choices. You are the same. It's time to break your food addiction and live a healthy lifestyle. I have come to find that people think that eating healthy is bland, boring and drab. It does not have to be. No one said you had to eat dry rice and raw broccoli. There are so many wonderful ways to eat healthy food. Once I turned my cooking skills into creatively preparing healthy dishes I was hooked. I fell in love with the bright colors of vegetable, the texture and the flavors. Remember that my companion e-book, "Clean Eating for People on the Go" is available as a resource too.

After working with countless of people, I have found that people disagree with this following statement: You are your top priority. Many feels as if their husband, family and children are their top priority. Men sometimes feel the same. They feel like their top priority is to provide income everyday only and not take care of their physical bodies. But is your body supposed to be unattended to and not cared for? Read this next statement slowly: YOU ARE IMPORTANT!

You are to love yourself and take care of yourself. That is not being selfish and one-sided. You need self-care. You need good health, a balanced energy level and you deserve to take care of yourself. You are beautiful. You are handsome. You can no longer put everything and everyone before your health and how you care for yourself. That is a recipe for disaster. You must find time every day to properly care for yourself. You deserve this. Technically, in caring for yourself you are caring for your family because they reap the benefits. They reap the reward of having a happier, healthier you. They reap the rewards of you having energy to run around the backyard and play catch. They get to hold unto the memory of how you would take a walk with them in the park without you becoming tired and needing to sit down for a quick rest.

Good health is not just for certain people; it's for everyone. Don't get into a negative frame of mind when it comes to looking at others. Clear your mind of these types of thoughts: "Well, she is just naturally thin, so she doesn't have to work that hard." Or, "He has time to go to the gym because he doesn't have kids." If you think like this, you are creating excuses as to why working out and being healthy is not right for you.

When you allow yourself to say you "cannot" do something, you are actually saying that you "will not" do it. Benjamin Franklin said, "You can do anything that you set your mind to" and I believe that. You need to believe that too. You need to believe that you can be healthy and maintain a healthy lifestyle on a consistent and on-going basis.

As a child and through my early adulthood, I struggled with low self-esteem. From being teased about how big my eyes were to being teased about how short I am, I developed an "I'm not good enough" attitude. I allowed the opinions of others to shape me and form the way that I looked at myself. I wanted to be accepted by others so badly that I became a "people pleaser". I didn't know my value and because of that I depended upon what others thought of me. I let them determine my worth. I didn't know that in trying to please others I was only hurting myself.

This low self-esteem crept into my outlook on my health. I didn't value myself. I didn't make myself a priority. I was one of those negative people that I just spoke of. Secretly, I was very critical of other women who were in good shape. To admit that I had thoughts of, "who does she think she is anyway?" would be the most transparent of transparencies. These thoughts were really revealing that I was jealous of those that were in good physical shape and good health. But the only reason that I was jealous is because I did not believe in myself and my low self-esteem issues kept me from seeing myself as to who I really was and how I could live my life. I didn't stop to think that I could be in good health and good shape too. The lesson to learn here is to use someone else's passion for eating healthy and exercising as a positive motivation to move you forward.

As I have repeatedly stated, good health is for everyone and once that light bulb turned on in my head I never looked back. Now as a result of my lifestyle change, I share my journey with others. Sharing my journey has been so rewarding.

Now that I lead a healthy lifestyle, people ask me quite often how do I maintain my weight loss? How did I overcome the fear of gaining back the weight? I also get asked quite often if I struggle with wanting to go back to my old habits?

The answer to these questions are that I put some safe guards in place for myself. I identified what my triggers were and I decided that I was not going to return to those poor habits. It's as simple as that. Once you condition your mind to not do something you just don't' do it.

Go back to the red-light analogy that I gave earlier in this book. We were taught in drivers training school that if we ran a red light there could be horrible repercussions, right? Like what? We could get a ticket. We could run into someone else or we could even get hit. Obviously, we do not want any of those things to happen so it just makes sense not to run a red light.

This same mindset is the mindset that I take that helps me to keep my weight off. For the year following me reaching my weight loss goals, I decided not to eat potato chips. I knew that if I returned to potato chips, I would gain back a good amount of weight. You might think this is too extreme but it wasn't. It was what I needed. It was my safe guard to make sure I stayed focused on my health and not gain back weight. I met my goal. I went a whole year without eating any potato chips at all.

You have the capability to change your life around too. I KNOW you can do it. Strength is yours and that strength will come out when you dig deep and muster the courage to stand by your decision that "enough is enough." Don't wait another moment. Don't procrastinate another day. Don't talk yourself out of living a healthy lifestyle. Take the first step today and watch how your life will change.

Just imagine how healthy you will feel by eating healthy on a consistent basis? Imagine wearing a smaller size dress. Envision the smile on your child's face when you have the energy to play football with them. Think about how great it will be to go up and down the stairs without huffing and puffing. These things, plus more, are waiting for you. It is time to take yourself off the "weight" list.

In the next five chapters, you will learn concepts as to how to live a consistent, healthy lifestyle. These concepts will help you not just for a week or to simply fit into your old wedding dress. These concepts can help you stay on the journey to good health for many years to come.

One More Thing

"Believe you can & you're halfway there."
T. Roosevelt

Interlude 4

Roxy in Desperation

Roxy woke up exhausted that morning but the smell of the coffee brewing in the kitchen brought hope. For the last 4 nights, she had been tossing and turning and unable to sleep. After meeting with her doctor, he gave her a list of things that she had to change in order to see positive changes in her life. Although coffee was high on the list she figured one more cup wouldn't hurt. Would it?

"Thanks for starting the coffee for me …That was so nice of you," said her husband as he interrupted her thoughts.

She turned around and looked at him standing there with the lifestyle change list from the doctor's office in his hand.

"You did turn that coffee pot on for me, right?"
"Uh, yes, sure I did. Why would I still be drinking coffee?"
"That's what I thought. That's my Angel face right there," as he planted a big, juicy kiss on her cheek.

Roxy's shoulders slumped as she turned on her heels and slowly walked to the couch. She had about 20 minutes before Chunky Boy usually starting stirring in his crib and would be wide awoke and ready to start his day.

With her husband now in the shower she was left alone.

She muttered to herself, "How did I end up like this? I didn't realize that my health was starting to fail me." Roxy picked up the new brightly-colored journal off the table. It was leather bound with a beautiful teal tassel to mark the day. Her and Charles even picked out a new pen for her too when they were at the office supply store.

Keeping a journal was something that Dr. Roman suggested to her when they met with him last week. He said that through writing she could express her emotions and face her fears. He said that research showed that those who journal have a higher chance of losing weight and keeping it off.

Roxy flipped through the blank pages of her new journal. She wasn't too sure about expressing her thoughts on paper; she never kept a diary before as a teenager so why should she start now? Still not quite sure that this would work for her, she thought to herself, "I guess I could give it a try. What I have been doing hasn't been working anyway considering how unhealthy I am."

On the 1st page of the book under "This book belongs to," she wrote in "Roxy...a woman who needs help."

9 TAKE ME OFF THE WEIGHT LIST

STEP 1: FORGIVE YOURSELF AND MOVE ON

Let's dive right in. How does forgiving yourself relate to weight loss? When you are mad at yourself because of your current state of health, you start to self-sabotage yourself. You have to forgive yourself for being in the current state that you are in. You have to consciously allow a new mindset to overtake your thinking. You can no longer think thoughts of "I'm already overweight so I might as well eat these cookies." You are no longer allowed to say "I'll never be in good shape, so what's the use?"

Merriam-Webster defines forgive as "to stop feeling angry towards and to stop blaming." Can you visualize being angry at yourself? Is it possible? Yes, it is possible and you might not even realize it.

Unforgiveness can materialize in so many ways. For me it had a physical effect. Even though at the untimely death of my mother we had a great relationship, the years preceding were tumultuous at best. For many years, I had a love-hate relationship with my mother. At times she was mean, demanding and insensitive and un-caring towards my needs. I was also, mean, demanding, insensitive and disrespecting to her. I used to have chronic back and shoulder pain. Ironically, it was during those same years that Mom and I were at

98

odds. The unforgiveness that I carried towards her had created tension in my body; I was in a very toxic state. Once we found neutral ground and found peace, I started noticing that my chronic pains subsided. Once I forgave her completely, my muscles relaxed. I finally had relief and I felt the difference in my exercising too. Harboring unforgiveness within yourself is not healthy at all. It could possibly be standing in the way of you maintaining a healthy way of living.

One of the best things that you could ever do to start the process towards forgiving yourself (or others) is to not dwell on the past. The past is the past. Accept what has led you to where you are and move on. Those past situations do not have to determine your current state of being. Don't be mad at yourself; don't harbor unforgiveness towards yourself especially.

Take a moment and grab several sheets of lined paper. Title the first sheet "Me...currently." Close your eyes and take five deep breathes. Write out how you currently feel about your nutritional level, your current physical state and your exercise habits. Write out any situations in your life that has caused you to eat emotionally. Maybe you don't deal with stress well so it causes you to eat when your emotions are high. Write out how you feel deep down inside about your inconsistencies. Write out everything that comes to mind about how you see yourself. Take as much time as you need and use another sheet of paper if you need to. After you have written everything out, read it again. Now fold it in half and begin to rip it up! That's right, rip that paper up to shreds. What have you just done? You have just symbolically dismantled the barriers in your life that have been holding you back. You have just destroyed your negative mindset. Gather all those pieces of paper and throw them away. Take them straight to the garbage can.

Now take out another sheet of paper. Title it "The New Me". Close your eyes and take five deep breathes again. Envision how you want to be. Open your eyes and begin to write. Write out how the new you will look. Are you full of energy and vitality? Are you in control of your eating? Are you able to walk briskly? Are you smiling more? Are you leaner? Fitter? Healthier? Do you have a tighter core? Are you feeling free from negative thoughts and behaviors? Are your emotions in check? Are you no longer craving sweets? Do you have good habits? Are you living a healthy, balanced lifestyle? Are you cooking healthy meals instead of eating out all the time? Keep writing until you feel like you have completely described every aspect of the new you.

Once you are done, read it again and determine that what you have just written is going to be the new you. This is a powerful sheet of paper. With this sheet of paper, you can now set a different brain path. This sheet of paper defines who you are. Not the past sheets that you ripped to shreds. This new sheet of paper is the new definition of who you are. Own your words and make them yours. Start to see yourself in a different manner. This is the new you.

You need to do one more thing. You need to write out several one-line affirmations from what you just wrote. It might look like this:

- I love myself.
- I accept myself.
- I am fearfully and wonderfully made in the image of God.
- I will not allow my emotions to dictate how and when I eat.
- I will be in good health.
- I will be in good shape.
- I will be fit.
- I am free to live life on a higher nutritional level.

Post these words on your refrigerator. Put them on the mirror in your bathroom. Put them in your car. Email them to yourself. Set them as a daily reminder on your phone. Print them on beautiful card stock and frame them.

Do whatever it takes to keep them as a visual reminder of the new you. This is an important step. It takes the brain at least 3 weeks or more to create a new brain pattern. Begin to rehearse your positive affirmations several times throughout the day to make them a part of you. Every time you find yourself slipping back into your old mindset, you need to pull out these words and say them. Every time you have a hard week at work and on Friday you want to self-medicate with a big bowl of ice cream and a spoon, pull out these words.

The days ahead of you are so bright and full of hope and positivity. You are emerging as a new person and that is fantastic.

One More Thing

"Dwelling on past bad decisions you've made only allows those decisions to keep defining you. Forgive yourself and move on." Mandy Hale

10 TAKE ME OFF THE WEIGHT LIST

STEP 2: ESTABLISH WHY YOU EXIST AND WHAT IS YOUR PURPOSE?

To wander around aimlessly in life without a goal, vision or purpose can be quite sad. To not know where you are going can lead you to being undetermined and haphazardly living life. Lack of direction can lead you to places that you never thought that you could end up at. It could lead you to hanging out with people that you thought you never would hang out with. It could have you doing things that you thought you never would do.

I bet you are probably thinking, "Why would statements like this be in a weight loss and nutritional book?" Statements like this are in my weight loss and nutritional book because when you value something, you take good care of it.

If you know the meaning and purpose of your life, you will do everything possible to stay healthy and maintain a balanced lifestyle. You need good health to support you as you work towards your life goals.

Stop for a moment and think about this: What is your purpose in life?

Are you moving towards that purpose? Are you living out that purpose? Are you healthy enough to carry this purpose out? Can you positively answer these questions?

We all need to have goals and visions. To know who you are and what your life is all about is so rewarding. To work towards goals and visions is a beautiful thing to wake up to every morning! Now per chance, you do not have your purpose figured out, let me help you. I cannot let you keep reading this book if you are walking around in a daze.

I have five questions for you to answer. Read them twice before you write in your answers.

What am I naturally good at?

_____

What do I enjoy doing?

_____

What could I do every day if I never got paid to do it?

_____

What have I taught others to do?

_____

What would my dream occupation be?

_____

Your answer to each question might look something like this:

1. I am naturally good at organizing events.
2. I enjoy putting on events.
3. Every day I could set-up training events.

4. I have taught others how to plan their training events for their employees.
5. My dream occupation would be as a contractor for small companies and set-up training sessions for their company to train their new employees on the company's policies and procedures.

With these five questions, you have just identified one of your purposes. Did you notice that I said that you have identified "one of your purposes"? Most people have more than one thing that they are naturally gifted to do. Repeat the exercise as many times as you want and you will be surprised at what you will discover about yourself.

When you feel as if you have completely exhausted all areas of yourself, lay out all your answers. Rate each set in order of your true passions on a scale of 1 to 10. You might find something you loved so much is actually just a hobby and not something that you thought you would love to do every day as a career. If such is the case, then it could potentially not be considered a foundational purpose of your life. You might even find the reverse. You might find that what you thought was a hobby could potentially be a true purpose. Even still you might find that what you wrote down could actually be combined. Step back and really look at everything that you wrote down.

Now let's make your vision statement. You need to bring yourself to life! After I did this exercise several times, here is my vision statement: *I am a person that is passionate about health and fitness and I will teach others how to live life with energy and vitality.*

Write out your vision statement here:

_____

_____

_____

What do you think about your vision statement? Does it speak to exactly who you are? You are pretty passionate, aren't you? Re-read your statement several times to let it sink in. You have a lot of life to live. Your upcoming days are going to be fantastic.

In returning to look at your health in light of your purpose, can your current level of health support your vision statement? What needs to happen to your health so you can fulfill what you wrote on the lines above? Do you need stronger legs if you are seeking to take clients on hiking tours? Do you need a tighter core because you want to teach others how to dance?

My vision statement empowers me every day. I get up every day and determine to live a healthy lifestyle because I need to fulfill my vision statement. The reality of it all is that if I had continued on with my addiction to potato chips, candy and cookies, I would be shortchanging myself on having the natural support I need to live out my purpose. The trade-off is not worth it. Wouldn't you agree?

If you want more out of life, then today is your day to acknowledge why you are here. Don't just sit there and watch others live their life. Live out your purpose and be sure to choose a healthy, balanced lifestyle to help you support reaching your goals and living out your vision statement. You have a lot of life inside of you! It's time to live and today is that day.

One More Thing

"You were put on this earth to achieve your greatest self, to live out your purpose, and to do it courageously." Dr. Steve Maraboli

11 TAKE ME OFF THE WEIGHT LIST

STEP 3: REDEFINE YOUR MINDSET TOWARDS FOOD AND WHY YOU EAT

Food is technically fuel for your body. The type of fuel that is chosen will determine the performance of your body. I am not a mechanic but I studied a lot about the damage that could occur when the wrong fuel is put inside a gas tank. Since engines work off the components in fuel, the wrong type of fuel can cause the engine to break down and stop working. One of the key things that I learned when studying fuel for cars is that if you ever put the wrong gas in your car, you should not turn the car on. When you do, the fuel starts running through the engine and starts poorly affecting the engine. Ultimately, it will start to lose power.

The electric fuel management system is alerted that something is wrong and your ignition timing and your fuel injection timing will be thrown off not knowing how to function. Fuel burns at different rates too. So, the spark plugs are looking for a certain speed of the fuel in order to ignite the engine. If the speed is too slow, there will either be a backfire or the engine could turn in the wrong direction. Either scenario could play out to incurring quite an expense to get that poor fuel out of the tank and to get things working properly again.

Source: http://bit.ly/2xHxV98

Just imagine that your body is that engine. What if it responded that quickly when you put the wrong "fuel" or in essence the wrong food in it? Could you imagine sputtering and panting throughout the day and running out of the energy that you need? You would be lethargic and incapable of performing your daily tasks.

If eating an apple pie would give you a blockage in your intestines, later that afternoon, I'm sure you would not eat it. If you knew that eating two cookies that were just 300 calories in total would lead to an extra 5lbs. of being overweight tomorrow, I'm sure you would not eat them.

Consider this: How could changing your habit of eating two cookies per day help you? Darren Hardy, editor of Success magazine talks about this concept in his book, Compound Effect. Just how many calories would not be consumed over a six-month period if those two cookies per day were not eaten? 300 calories per day from January 1st to July 1st would be an estimate of 175 days. 175 days x 300 calories equal 52,500 calories. It only takes a deficient of 1,200 calories to lose one pound. Approximately 43lbs. could potentially be shredded off of your body if you refrained from eating two cookies per day. Although this cookie calorie count is hypothetical, it might be worth dropping that bedtime cookie ritual.

To dig further into resetting your mindset into the true purpose of food, I briefly touched on my connection to food and those delicious, warm cinnamon rolls that my Mom used to make our family. In observing my Mom, she made these rolls when she was in a happy mood. They were a lot of work for her to make but when she made them, she was "in the mood" to make them. I naturally grew up thinking that you baked sweet treats when you were in a happy mood. I found that I continued on in life I would eat from my emotions, at both happy times and ultimately at sad times as well. What kind of emotional connections have you made with food?

When food is being used in its proper use, you will make balanced calculated decisions on what you are eating and not eat because of a situation or an emotion. To eat when you are happy, sad, angry or stressed out could possibly land you in the range of overeating when your emotions are heightened. Your mind is far from thinking about what food groups you are eating to determine if it is a healthy meal or not. You should be eating to live vs. living to eat.

So, how do you control your emotions to reduce emotional eating?

1. Be present in the moment. When I am faced with a situation, I embrace that current situation and let the emotion be controlled and self-contained. I no longer run away from it or look for an outlet through eating. I stay present in that situation and deal with whatever is going on right then and there.

2. Have a level and even mindset. To acknowledge that all situations have a resolution is a large statement, I know. If you stay in a state of being level-minded, you are more apt to be rational and calm when situations come about. Learn to be in control of yourself vs. letting someone else control you and your responses.

3. Play by the rules. If your whole life is dependent upon Jesus Christ and you follow the principles in the Bible that address being anxious for nothing, there is no room for being led by emotions. For me personally, casting my cares upon Jesus has totally and completely revamped my life.

Learn to use food in its proper use and you will see great results in your health.

One More Thing

"Food is more than a matter of taste, it is the fuel for our bodies." Jane Fonda

12 TAKE ME OFF THE WEIGHT LIST
STEP 4: CREATE A NEW YOU

Everywhere we turn we are faced with the phraseology of "creating a new you." I've even said it a couple of times in this book. It seems like every magazine in the checkout lane has a title that confirms that too. Have we as a society become vain and obsessed with ourselves? The answer to that question is both "yes" and "no". There are people who never focus on themselves...ever. Why is that? Why do some people feel that it is all about them and others shy away and cringe at the thought of doing anything that will take attention away from their spouse or their children? I briefly touched on focusing on yourself in chapter 9 but I want to expand on the topic here a little further.

Over the years that I have been a health coach, I have come across countless people who simply felt that they are not important. They seem to have the mindset that to focus on themselves with a few minutes of exercising will make them conceded and self-absorbed and only looking out for themselves. On the contrary, there is nothing wrong with valuing yourself enough and doing something positive for yourself so you can look and feel great.

While I am not a psychologist or have never studied in that field, I am

110

able to detect when people do everything for others and put others before themselves. I need to be transparent because I am a perfect example of that.

I had a lot of responsibility as a teenager. I took care of my family and my two younger brothers. I am 12 years older than my middle brother and 14 years older than my youngest brother. Whenever I wanted to go out and play with my friends, I had to take my brothers with me. While you might not think that was the worst thing in the world let me paint a broader picture. I washed their clothes and I groomed them. I read to them. I told them everything would be ok when they were scared. I did not get a chance to focus on myself because all I knew to do was to focus on my brothers and my family.

As a married woman, I found this same trend continuing. My husband and I got married when we were 23. Young love! We had our two boys at the beginning our marriage. With deciding to raise our boys at home, I soon became a stay-at-home mother. I was at home with them for 14-1/2 years. I poured my life out into our family, holding nothing back and being there at their every beck and call. It was an honor to have such a responsibility.

Along with that responsibility came the realization that I very rarely paid myself any attention and with that came on the low self-esteem issues and the weight gain. I got stuck on an emotional roller coaster that I could not get off of. On days that I tried to focus on myself, it seemed like something went lacking. Either dinner was late or my boys did not get put down for their nap on time and my schedule was thrown off. I would back off of whatever I was doing for myself.

I finally woke up in 2015 and decided that it was time for me to focus on myself. I combined a healthy dose of being a little vain and a much-deserved focus on myself. What about you? Have you been lost in your rhythm of life and have lost sight on focusing on yourself? You are important and you matter.

Use these three mindsets to reclaim some much-needed self-awareness:

1. Appreciate who you are. You are your own person. You have your own set of skills, talents and abilities. You have your own personality and characteristics. Accept that. You are different and you are unique. Be comfortable with who you are. Celebrate you.
2. Do not compare yourself to others. To size yourself up to someone else just does not make any sense. You have no clue what they went through to get to where they are. To wish that you could be like them might be wishing a life of hurt, pain and misery upon yourself. Be careful what you wish for. Be grateful for what you have.
3. Believe in yourself. You deserve to have time to focus on you. You are worth it!

I have another daily affirmation that I use to remind me of who I am and how valuable I am. Through it I shape my emotions, my outlook on life and my levels of health and fitness. My daily affirmation reminds me that I am important and that it is ok to focus on me.

I am an accomplished and successful woman. I deserve to take time out of my daily schedule to focus on me. I will use my food as fuel and I will not over eat. I am in good shape and I will have good health. I will live a consist and balanced lifestyle. I love myself enough to take care of me!

Now it's your turn. While answering the following questions as a guideline, create your daily affirmation statement. Use the space below to craft your affirmation.

1. What negative mindsets do you need to let go of in order to reach your goals?
2. What health and fitness goals would you like to achieve?
3. What fears do you need to face in regards to feeling guilty when it comes to caring for yourself?
4. What do you need to rearrange in your schedule to create time for yourself?

Guidelines for writing your affirmations: Think positive. Write your affirmations in terms of how you would like your life to be. Write from the aspect of seeing yourself as completing your goals. Paint your future. Ready, set, go!

_____

_____

_____

To make these affirmation statements a part of your life, just like you did with your vision statement in chapter 10, you need to read them out loud to yourself daily. Doing this will help you envision yourself just as you would like to be. When you talk positive, you think positive and when you think positive, positive things happen. Change your life today and start talking positively!

Here are a few other places where you can make your affirmation accessible and readable on a daily basis.

1. Put it on your bathroom mirror.
2. Put it in a picture frame by your bed.
3. Save it as your desktop background on your computer.
4. Read them into a recorder and play them back to yourself each day.

Get creative and find a special place to put your affirmation. You should read your affirmation statements out loud and on an everyday basis. Once again, remember that daily rehearsing of your affirmation will cause your mindset to line up with your desires for how you want to be. Your actions will then follow.

Practice right now. Stand in front of a mirror. Read your affirmation statements out loud. Say it like you mean it. Repeat it again. You are on your way to the new you!

One More Thing

"We can't become what we need to be by remaining what we are." Oprah

---

13 TAKE ME OFF THE WEIGHT LIST
STEP 5: ACCOUNTATBILITY IS KEY

In turning our full attention to remaining on the path to good health and nutrition, let's look at ways to instill accountability. A lack of discipline has been the biggest culprit for people who struggle with maintaining a consistent, healthy lifestyle.

Accountability is a big scary word that people seem to run from. Believe it or not, we already have accountability in our everyday lives. If you have a job, your boss expects you to come to work at a certain time. If you have children, they count on you to pick them up from school and feed them dinner. If you own a business, your customers expect you to ship out their orders once they pay you for them.

These are all daily situations where you are to be accountable, right? So why shortchange yourself on your health? Don't take a gamble on your health, it's not worth it.

Your body is dependent upon you. It is so important to be accountable to yourself.

115

Lack of accountability can lead to a vicious cycle. For example, a lack of accountability in eating healthy could lead to yo-yo dieting.

The Cycle of Yo-Yo Dieting

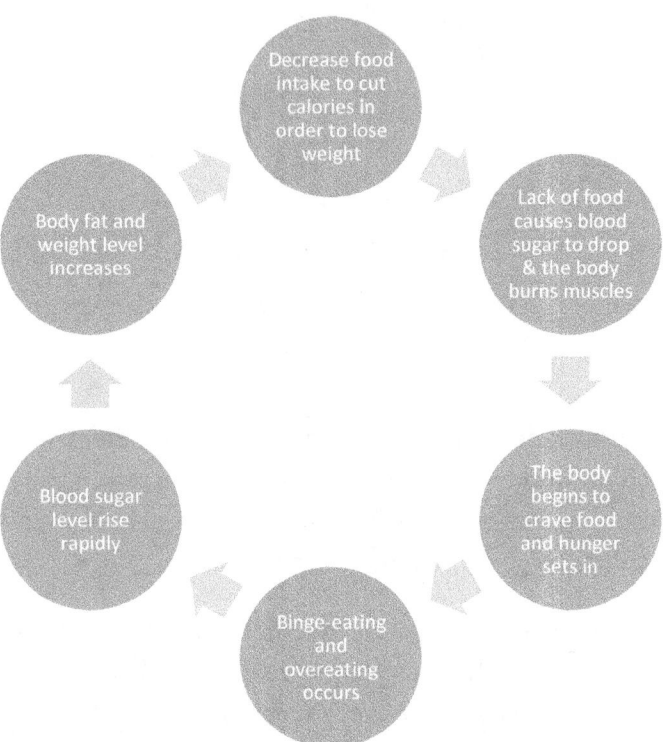

The best way to end this cycle is to stop it before it even begins. Any type of drastic cut in calories to lose weight is an absolute no-no unless you are cutting empty calories. If you are a regular pop drinker or Frappuccino drinker and you cut out those calories, then you are on the right path. But if you decide to stop eating 500 calories less altogether just to lose weight, you are more than likely sacrificing some nutrients that you need. You will be throwing off your metabolism and you will be losing muscle weight to which is dangerous.

If you are ready to break the cycle of being unaccountable, try one of these methods to help you get on track:

1. Let a friend know what your health and fitness goals are or write them out and give them to your friend. Ask them to check in with you daily or weekly.

2. Tell your children your goals. Children have an incredible sense of memory. (Just think about the last time you promised them something and you didn't do it!) If you tell your child to ask you daily about your goals when you pick them up from school, you will be forced to be held accountable.

3. Grab a calendar. Write down your goal each day of the week. Cross off each time that you actually meet your goal and celebrate your accomplishment!

4. Hire a health and fitness coach. I know all too well the first-hand success stories that I have seen with my clients. I am 100% committed to all of my clients and I am accessible 24-7. Clients that rely heavily on me have seen amazing results. Why is that? I am encouraging them and motivating them to succeed. I celebrate right along with them when they reach their goal of drinking water for the day or when they eat all their servings of vegetables for the day or when they go down a pants size. These are all the benefits of hiring Health Coach Shalynne.

You might say these things are easier said than done, right? There might be some truth to that. But, these ideas will work for you when you are 100% committed to yourself. You have to believe in yourself.

You are capable of being so much more than what you give yourself credit for. You are capable of making sound decisions and sticking with them. Good health is for all! There is nothing wrong with taking time out of each day to do something good for yourself. You deserve to take care of yourself. You are one amazing person who is full of gifts and talents. You have awesome skills and talents. Clear away the self-doubt that having good health is not for you. Stop second guessing yourself as to "if" you can achieve your health and fitness goals. You can and you will! Why else did you buy this book if you didn't believe that about yourself? Today is a great day to start your journey to accountability. You can do it. I believe in you. Your best days are right around the corner.

One More Thing

"It is not only what we do, but also what we do not
do for which we are accountable."
John Baptiste Moliere

14 HOW TO HANDLE DISTRACTIONS AND HOW TO RUN FROM DONUTS

What does it take to live a life based upon your health and fitness goals? How do you survive in a world full of fast food restaurants on every other corner? How do you pass up all the candy and treats in the checkout line? Do you feel like you are set-up for failure with how easy it is to pick up a café latte at the nearest coffee shop? And why are so many delicious things loaded with trans-fat and addictive addends like sugar?

Here is my humorous Survivor's Guide on How to Pass Up Junk Food:

1. Walk in the holiday party and flip the dessert table over!

2. Carry a bull horn and every time someone offers you junk food scream in their ear, "Please back away from me. I cannot eat junk food."

3. Wear a blindfold when you go grocery shopping.

4. Strap on 50lbs. of lard to your waist to remind you how much weight you could potentially gain when you eat junk food.

119

5. Embed sensors in your tongue so every time you eat sweets, your tongue pushes the food out.

6. Put hot sauce drips into your fingertips so that hot sauce squirts out whenever you touch junk food.

7. Hire a bagpipe marching band to follow you around 24-7 and tell them to play a very annoying song when you order dessert at a restaurant.

8. Put radars in your head so that when you think about eating the Halloween candy that your kids bring home that you instantly get dizzy and fall over.

9. Put skunk fragrance in your nose hairs so you can no longer smell a fresh batch of chocolate chip cookies.

10. Put springs in your butt so that every time you sit down to eat a huge bowl of ice cream you instantly spring into the air and out the roof.

Ok...so let's be serious! Here is my true Survivors Guide on How to Pass up Junk Food.

De-Junk yourself, Option One:

Eat before you go to the party. If you show up at the party and your stomach is growling, then you have set yourself up for utter disaster. You will eat everything in sight and you will be just like a bear with no restraints. Have a small snack of nuts, apple and a type of protein like chicken, boiled egg or turkey bacon before you leave. These foods will help curve your appetite. You will be more apt to eat in moderation with an underlying layer of food in your stomach. When you get to the party do not run in through the door and push people out of the way screaming, "Food! I need food!". You should actually be the last in line. What?!?! Yes, I said you should be last in line. Before you slam this book closed, let me explain…. please. When you really think about it, what food goes first at a party? All the foods that are loaded with heavy butters, creams, and sugar. That would be the macaroni and cheese, the yams and probably the lasagna with garlic bread. What do you think are the main types of dishes that people leave on the table? Yup! You guessed it. All the healthy foods: the salads, vegetables and other sugar free dishes. Who wants to eat that??? That's right. You do! When you want to eat healthy, you have to do things differently. Next time be the last in line.

De-Junk Yourself, Option 2:

<u>Don't go to the grocery store without a shopping list…ever</u>: Going to the grocery store without a shopping list is like walking into hell without a glass of water. Oops! Not sure if that will be edited out but I'll give it a try. It's a perfect analogy, isn't it? First of all, no one wants to go to hell and no one wants to be caught in hell without anything cold to drink. It is the exact same thing that will happen when you go to the grocery store unprepared. Your cart is going to be full of stuff that you think you need but you really do not need. The question remains then: How do you know what groceries you really need? How do you plan and ward off this dangerous act in the making?

Here's the two-step process:

Step 1: Plan out your meals for the week. Take a Friday afternoon or Saturday morning to plan out what you want to eat for the upcoming week. What about breakfast? Is it easier to make a healthy loaf of banana nut bread and serve an apple with it? Or, maybe have a quick bowl of oatmeal with nuts and raisins? Put it on the list. How do you set-up lunches? Do you put money in your budget for a quick lunch at the cafe two days a week or will you carry a salad every day and just need to buy snack packages of nuts for the ride home? And what about dinner? Will you have spaghetti one night and baked chicken another? Will you eat dinner out on Thursday because one of the kids has a late practice and there will be no time to cook dinner after work? Take the time to stop and take an overview of the week ahead and determine how many meals you will need to eat and what dishes you want to cook. Once you have everything all planned out, take your list to your kitchen and determine what items you are missing. Make your list from there and then you can safely head out to the store.

Step 2: If at all possible leave the kids at home! Ok, spoken like a true empty nester on my part, right? I know you like the oo's and ah's that you get from taking your cute little 3-year-old into the grocery store with you, but how hard is it to say "no" to that cute little face when they are begging you for those cookies that are not on your grocery list? And, do not forget about the candy bars that are right at the kid level when you get to the counter to pay. If at all possible, leave the kids at home. They will entice you to put things in your shopping cart that you did not intend to be in there. If unplanned for items makes it to your house guess who is going to be sitting down to eat those things with that cute little 3-year-old? Yup, you guessed it.

De-Junk Yourself, Option 3:

Reward yourself with dessert once a week: What is the fun of having a great lifestyle of eating healthy if you cannot splurge every once in a while? How do you plan a splurge anyway? I pick a day of the week when I know I am going to most enjoy my hard-earned treat. For me, it's Friday. There is something about working hard all week at work. On Friday's I just want to kick back and wolf down my snack. Let's put this in perspective though. I am not talking about eating a whole pan of brownies and a whole tub of ice cream. Come on...this is a weight loss book, right? I'm taking about a brownie square with a good dollop of ice cream. Sounds reasonable, right? Who wouldn't want to work to earn the thing that they love to eat? I work hard every week for my snack. Pick your snack and pick your day and set yourself up for success and not failure. Utilize the 80/20 rule that I talked about in chapter 5. Remember, following this rule will help steer your health to a manageable and balanced way of consistent, healthy living.

De-Junk Yourself, Option 4:

Keep the junk food for the rest of the family in a separate locked container to which you do not have a key. (Smile)

Ok, I know this sounds extreme too but hear me out. As you know, my addiction was to potato chips. This was a true addiction to the point where I would be in another part of the house and I would hear the potato chips calling my name. I swear this is the truth! Locking food away was the first step to breaking my addiction. Truth be told, I did not have a chest with a padlock on it, but the potato chips were in a separate place. There is truth to: "Out of sight, out of mind!" I literally separated the snacks for my children and husband from my snacks. This was extremely effective because when I opened up the pantry all I saw were options that I could just reach right in and eat. Try it. It really works!

Putting these steps into practice will help you learn to control your selection in choice of food. And just like the name of this chapter states, you have now learned how to run from donuts!

One More Thing

"Don't ask why healthy food is so expensive. Ask
why junk food is so cheap."
Nutrition Snob

Interlude 5

Roxy in Determination

It had been 3 weeks since Charles bought Roxy a gym membership at 1, 2, 3: Fitness is For Me. With over 100 locations across Charleston, he knew that it would be easy for her to drop in for a workout session whenever she needed it. Especially with them having on-site childcare they felt that they made the right choice for her. She was worth that and more. He just couldn't understand why she had only been once so far. He had been trying to support her and encourage her to go to the gym but he could tell that she wasn't in the mood to exercise after her long days of working, cooking dinner, cleaning the house and taking care of Chunky Boy.

"What could I do to support her more?" he said to himself as he sat at his desk at work. "I know. I could go with her. Maybe that would help."

He pulled out his cell phone and sent a text.

"Hey. You there?"
"Hi. What's up?" came the reply.
"I have an idea. What if I go with you to the gym?"

Roxy stared at the text message and felt a glimmer of hope. How did he realize that that was her biggest fear? She hadn't even told him that yet. But going to the gym alone was so scary. She immediately thought about how she felt when she went last week for the first time.

The bright lights. The loud music. The damp, lingering smell of sweat and all the people who already had great shapes stared at her immediately as she walked in. She even remembered how intimidated she was getting on the treadmill for the first time. She almost fell off and quickly pulled the emergency cord for it to stop. Such a disaster. If it wasn't for the nice lady who saw her struggling, she would have run out the gym.

"I would like that." She texted back.

With only being married for 8 years and comfortably fitting in her wedding dress on her wedding day, Roxy would never have imagined that in such a short amount of time she could be 45lb. overweight and have diabetes. Although she realized that she was starting to breathe rather heavy when she would have to go to the basement to do the laundry, she wanted to look past that warning sign that something greater was happening to her health.

Roxy put her cell phone back on her desk and decided to take a break.

"Trina, I'm stepping away for a minute," Roxy said to the floor secretary.
Trina nodded in acknowledgement since she was on a call at the time.

Roxy walked past a sea of grey cubicles and followed the path to the only ladies' restroom on the 5th floor. She worked hard to become a mid-level Customer Service manager at Twilight, a wholesale supplier of nighttime eyewear. She would have never dreamed that she could make that type of money with coming from a family where she was the first to graduate from college.

Roxy opened the bathroom door and noticed that all the stalls were empty. She walked up to the 3rd mirror and just stood there. With a great job, a beautiful baby and a supportive husband, why was she so unhappy with the image in the mirror? Didn't she have a lot to be grateful for?

Until that very moment, she hadn't realized how round her face had gotten. What had she done to herself? A tear slowly slides down her face.

Roxy brushed the tear off her face and said, "It is time."

15 WHERE DO I GO FROM HERE?

Welcome to the back of the book! The best thing that you ever did to help along your current nutritional state is to pick up this book. The next best thing that you did is to read this book in its entirety. Congratulations!

The logical question now is, "Where do you go from here?" You have learned to follow a new way of thinking. You now have foundational truths about health based upon biblical scripture. You are now equipped with educational health facts and concepts. The last step is to put it all together.

My intent in writing this book was to help you realize your potential. To realize that you are capable of living a consistent, healthy lifestyle without all the ups and downs and the yo-yo way of eating. Why deal with the stress of constantly worrying about your weight? Having to take pills to control your high blood pressure or having 3 to 5 different sizes of clothes in your closet?

I personally know how hard it is being attached to food mentally and emotionally and being controlled by its dictating powers. I know how you feel when you are alone in the car and in a split second, you pull into the drive through lane and order some food. In that moment, your mind plays tricks on you to make you think that it is easier to pick up something instead of spending 35 minutes to cook a healthy meal when you get home because you are beyond tired.

Today is the dawning of a new day for you. Your opportunity to make some changes is here. This is your defining moment to determine how you really want to live. *You* get to choose how healthy *you* want to be. Go back through this book and follow the principles that were laid out for you. Apply them to your life. When you change your mindset, you will see a dramatic change in your health.

Today is your day to say, "Take me off the weight list."